NAVIGATING THE BOARDROOM

40 Maxims - Things You Must Know and
Do to Be a Great Director

By:

Dennis D. Pointer

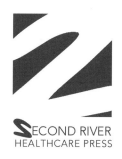

SECOND RIVER
HEALTHCARE PRESS

NAVIGATING THE BOARDROOM
40 Maxims
Things You Must Know and Do to Be a Great Director

Second River Healthcare Press
26 C Shawnee Way
Bozeman, MT 59715

Phone (406) 586-8775
FAX (406) 586-5672

Editor: Michelle Nash
Cover Design: Christopher R. Jackson
Cover Art: Lan Weisberger
Typesetting/Composition: Shore Design

Pointer, Dennis NAVIGATING THE BOARDROOM: 40 Maxims – Things You Must Know and Do to Be a Great Director / Dennis D. Pointer

ISBN-10: 0-9743860-9-X   ISBN-13: 978-0-9743860-9-6

1. Board of Directors   2. Hospital Trustees   3. Governance

Library of Congress Control Number: 2008927071

First Printing   May 2008

For ordering information regarding Second River Healthcare Press books, please call (406) 586-8775 or visit the website:

www.SecondRiverHealthcare.com

ABOUT THE AUTHOR

Dennis D. Pointer, Ph.D. is Austin Ross – Virginia Mason Professor, Department of Health Administration, School of Public Health and Community Medicine, University of Washington (Seattle). He has held two previous endowed chairs: John J. Hanlon Professor of Health Services, Graduate School of Public Health, San Diego State University (1991-2002); and Arthur Graham Glasgow Professor of Health Services Management, Department of Health Administration, Medical College of Virginia, Virginia Commonwealth University (1986-1991). From 1975 to 1986 he was affiliated with the University of California - Los Angeles where he served as: Professor and Head, Program in Health Services Management, School of Public Health; Associate Director, U.C.L.A. Medical Center; Professor, Anderson School of Management; and Professor of Psychiatry and Bio-behavioral Sciences, School of Medicine. During his tenure at U.C.L.A. he was a Research Fellow at the RAND Corporation. He has held faculty appointments at the Mount Sinai School of Medicine (New York) and the Baruch School of Management of the City University of New York in addition to having served as Associate Director, Department of Teaching Hospitals, Association of American Medical Colleges (Washington, D.C.).

Denny is the author of eleven books. *Really Governing* and *Board Work* have won the James A. Hamilton Book of the Year Award from the American College of Healthcare Executives. His other books include: *Getting to Great: Principles of Health Care Organization Governance*; *The High-Performance Board: Principles of Nonprofit Organization Governance*; *The Health Care Industry: A Primer for Board Members*; *Essentials of Health Care Organization Finance: A Primer for Board Members*; and *Governing the 21st Century Nonprofit Healthcare Organization: Transforming the Work and Contributions of Your Board* (in process; estimated release in early 2009). He has written 80 scholarly and professional articles.

Principal of Dennis D. Pointer & Associates, Denny has been

retained as a governance consultant, retreat facilitator and speaker by over 250 healthcare organizations, commercial corporations, governmental agencies and professional/trade associations. He was a founding partner of the American Healthcare Governance and Leadership Group LLC, now the Center for Healthcare Governance of the American Hospital Association.

Denny received his Ph.D. from the University of Iowa in hospital and health services administration and B.Sc. in organizational psychology from Iowa State University.

LETTER TO READERS

Dear Colleagues:

There are approximately 10,000 nonprofit healthcare provider organization boards in the U.S., each of which has about 15 members. Thus, the best-guess number of directors is 150,000.

The effectiveness of these boards...the extent they make a difference on behalf of their communities and add value to the organizations they govern...depends on the qualities of directors: their dedication, effort, knowledge, skills, experience and perspectives. Although governing is a "team sport," it's practiced by individuals who occupy all those boardroom chairs.

The vast governance literature has focused almost exclusively on boards: their obligations, responsibilities and roles; the way they should be structured, configured and composed; how they should function; and what they can do to improve their performance. Little attention has been accorded directors and directorship. This book was written to begin filling that void.

Drivers' manuals aren't provided to directors at the time of their initial appointment or during their terms of service. The assumption is that bright people will figure out, and pick up the fundamentals of, board work by just doing it. While experience *is* a great teacher, it can be enriched, leveraged and enlivened when grounded on good ideas.

> *max•im* (mac'sîm); Succinct formulation of a fundamental principle; a guideline for thinking, deciding and acting.

Navigating the Boardroom forwards 40 maxims, some things you must know and do to maximize your performance and contributions as a nonprofit healthcare organization director, whether you're new or long-tenured. The book is straight talk that forwards practical and usable wisdom.

This is a product of what I've learned over 30 years of governance consulting, teaching, research, writing and speaking. I've spent a huge amount of time in boardrooms with directors, both colleagues and clients. I owe these folks a large debt; they are, in every sense, my co-pilots in this endeavor (bearing none of the blame for what you might find ill-conceived or poorly stated). Additionally, it has been my good fortune to have worked with a bunch of wonderful collaborators/friends over the years. With trepidations regarding sins of omission, thanks to (in alphabetical order): Gary Aden, Ted Ball, Jim Begun, Rick Carlson, David Cohen, John Colloton, Bill Dowling, Charlie Ewell, Debbie Gramling, Leo Greenawalt, Jan Jennings, Nate Kaufman, Dick Knapp, Jennifer Kozakowski, Baldwin Lamson, Sam Levey, Roice Luke, Michele Molden, Jerry Norville, Jamie Orlikoff, Andy Pasternack, Dave Pitts, Jerry Pogue, Austin Ross, Marty Ross, Lou Rossiter, Bob Simmons, Mary Totten, Tim Stack, Dennis Stillman, Will Welton and Steve Williams...you've all enriched my life.

I wanted to keep this book short. [Maye West was wrong when she said, "Too much of a good thing is great."] So, rather than including numerous referenced supplemental materials as appendices, they're provided at www.BoardFood.com; go to the *navigation aids, other resources* or *bookshelf pages* and download what you find useful/interesting. The website also contains a "truck-load" of other governance "knowledgeware," all provided as open-source documents.

Denny
Dennis D. Pointer
Seattle, Washington
dpointer@u.washington.edu

REVIEWS

"All directors should read these 40 Maxims; they will change the way you think about governing and the way you perform in the boardroom"

Douglas Hawthorne
President & CEO
Texas Health Resources
Arlington, TX

"Denny has a nose for understanding best practices and worst mistakes. He lays out 'rules of the road' for novice and experienced directors alike. Everyone who enters a health system or hospital boardroom can benefit from this book."

J. Knox Singleton
President & CEO
Inova Health System
Falls Church, VA

"An extraordinary book, very well written. The 40 maxims are right on target and valuable guides for all trustees. This is a must read."

Stephen A. Williams
President & CEO
Norton Healthcare
Louisville, KY

"I have spent 27 years of my life as the CEO of healthcare organizations, a publicly traded company and a start-up IT venture; I've always sought Denny's counsel and advice about governance. These maxims will help directors make good boards great. In an era of transparency, boards that heed these ideas will outshine their counterparts and be of greater value to society."

R. Timothy Stack
President & CEO
Piedmont Healthcare
Atlanta, GA

"CEOs are realizing strong, informed and empowered boards are great assets for navigating the challenges facing contemporary healthcare organizations. High performance governance requires: boards that engage in best practices; and directors who understand and execute their critical roles. Denny's book provides an essential road map for executives, board chairs and directors."

Gary S. Kaplan, M.D.
Chairman & CEO
Virginia Mason Medical
Center
Seattle, WA

"Denny has produced an invaluable guide about the self-care and development of board officers and members. It is targeted perfectly. I wish such a list of do's and don'ts had been available when I entered the field in 1955. Clearly, in today's complex environment, his contribution is of special value. It serves as a powerful guide to strengthen executive-board relationships."

Austin Ross
Executive Vice President,
Emeritus
Virginia Mason Medical
Center
Seattle, WA

TABLE OF CONTENTS

ABOUT THE AUTHOR

LETTER TO READERS

REVIEWS

MAXIM 1 Governance matters. 1

MAXIM 2 Evaluate your interest in, and commitment to, 3
the organization before serving or
continuing to serve.

MAXIM 3 Don't be a "letterhead" director. 5

MAXIM 4 Become a professional director. 7

MAXIM 5 Know what's expected of you. 9

MAXIM 6 Get to know your colleagues. 12

MAXIM 7 If you are a newly appointed director, 14
hook up with a mentor.

MAXIM 8 Immediately begin acquiring an understanding 17
of governance and the nature of board work.

MAXIM 9 Understand board topography. 19

MAXIM 10 Serve your apprenticeship, but do so quickly. 22

MAXIM 11 Realize governing is a distinctive 24
organizational practice.

MAXIM 12 Recognize the difference between governing 26
and managing, then respect it.

MAXIM 13 Keep your eyes on the prize. 29

MAXIM 14 Don't represent narrow interests or constituencies. 32

MAXIM 15 Understand your legal fiduciary duties of loyalty, 35
care and obedience in addition to director
liabilities/protections.

MAXIM 16 Understand your board's governing 41
responsibilities.

MAXIM 17 Acquire an increasingly sophisticated 47
understanding of content areas underpinning
issues your board will be addressing.

MAXIM 18 Develop (or enhance) your healthcare 51
organization-specific financial literacy.

MAXIM 19 If you're the board chair, learn how to run 55
effective and efficient meetings.

MAXIM 20 Do your homework. 58

MAXIM 21 Show up. 60

MAXIM 22 Participate. 62

MAXIM 23 Question. 65

MAXIM 24 Play devil's advocate. 67

MAXIM 25 Acknowledge conflicts-of-interests and disengage 69
when you have one.

MAXIM 26 Keep sensitive information confidential. 72

MAXIM 27 Be ethical. 75

MAXIM 28 Do governing work only in the boardroom. 79

MAXIM 29 Stroke. 81

MAXIM 30 Don't make individual requests of the CEO 82
and executive team members.

MAXIM 31 Be prepared to vote no. 84

MAXIM 3 2 Argue in the boardroom, lock arms 86
when you leave it.

MAXIM 3 3 Don't engage in personal financial dealings 87
with other directors or executives.

MAXIM 3 4 Never do non-governance work for the 90
organization.

MAXIM 3 5 Keep your personal relationship with the 92
CEO at arms-length.

MAXIM 3 6 Provide the CEO with advice and counsel, but be 94
careful.

MAXIM 3 7 Be prepared to lead. 96

MAXIM 3 8 Be a good board and organizational citizen. 98

MAXIM 3 9 Prior to the conclusion of each term, assess 99
your performance and contributions.

MAXIM 4O Enjoy the journey and have fun. 101

REFERENCES AND RESOURCES 105

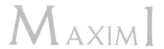MAXIM 1
GOVERNANCE MATTERS.

Healthcare organizations are important institutions. They're a critical part of your community's infrastructure, provide services affecting its wellbeing and have a significant economic impact.

"A board is as high up in an organization as one can go and still remain inside it" (from *Boards that Make a Difference*, by John Carver). Accordingly, your board bears ultimate responsibility and accountability for the organization: everything it is, does and should become; stewardship of its resources and capacities; and how well it serves your community.

Because your board is where the buck stops, its work has a potentially huge impact on the organization's performance and success. The issues your board addresses, and decisions it makes regarding them, defines the organization and shapes its future.

If you don't buy the notion that boards make a difference, consider this "reverse angle" thought experiment: Your board has 15 minutes to make decisions that would really harm the organization... strategically, managerially, financially, operationally or clinically. Could you do it? Every board to which I have posed this question has responded: "Yes, we're up to the challenge, it would be easy and wouldn't take 15 minutes." Your board, the work it does and how well it's done has a significant impact ... for better or worse.

Directorship

- Some contend that boards don't make a great deal of difference or add much value. They say: Directors are amateurs lacking a sophisticated understanding of the healthcare industry, local markets, community needs, competitors and the organizations they're governing. They also argue: The few things boards do reasonably well could

1

be done far better by management and physician leaders; boards just get in the way and slow down an organization's metabolism. What do you think? What value can boards add that executives and physician leaders can't? What are the distinctive purpose and contributions of boards? These questions are fundamental ones, to which I will return later.

- What difference does your board make and how much value does it add? During the past year, what were your board's most important contributions?

- In what ways has your board been a drag on the organization?

- What are some things that have inhibited/impaired your board from maximizing its performance and contributions?

- What do you bring to this boardroom; knowledge, skills, experiences and perspectives? How much of a contribution do you make?

- What are things you might do to become a better director?

M AXIM 2

EVALUATE YOUR INTEREST IN, AND COMMITMENT TO, THE ORGANIZATION BEFORE SERVING OR CONTINUING TO SERVE.

Being a high performing/contributing director requires considerable time and effort. Personal interest in issues being dealt with by the board should capture your attention and personal commitment to the organization's mission should sustain your involvement over the long haul. Both interest and commitment are necessary ingredients for great directorship.

Anecdote: Several years ago a colleague of mine resigned from a board she had joined only 14 months earlier. This board was first-rate and appointment to it was an honor. She had wanted to work with its members, all "movers and shakers." Additionally, its quarterly meetings provided her an opportunity to spend time with the CEO, a good friend. The problem, recognized too late: This organization's mission and issues the board addressed weren't important to her. Don't make a similar mistake.

Directorship

- How invested are you in this organization? What about it is really important to you? How committed are you to its vision and mission? How interested are you in issues passing through the boardroom?

- Why did you decide to join this board?

- Overall, how does this director/board experience stack up with others you've had?

- What would cause you to resign?

MAXIM 3

DON'T BE A "LETTERHEAD" DIRECTOR.

Being nominated or re-appointed to a healthcare organization board is an honor and privilege; recognizing you're a community leader and respected person in the eyes of your peers, plus offering you the opportunity to do important work and make a difference.

Letterhead directors are those who want the glory that comes with board membership but rarely attend meetings and don't participate or contribute much. There are several good reasons, beyond the obvious ones, for not being this type of director:

- It totally depreciates the value associated with board membership you wanted when signing on.

- You're accountable and potentially liable for board decisions/actions, even when you don't attend meetings. Indeed, you breach the fiduciary duty of care (see *Maxim #15*) through non-attendance and participation.

- By taking a seat and then "checking out," you rob the board of a valuable asset.

Serve, and continue serving, because you have something to contribute and are willing/able to do so.

Directorship

- In all communities, the pool of talented/connected leaders is small and such folks are sought by many organizations to serve on their boards. Your interest, time and effort are finite and you have a wide variety of opportunities for giving something back. Why did you choose this board as a way of making a contribution?

- On how many boards do you presently serve? If it's more than three, evaluate if you're spread too thin.

- If you no longer have the necessary time or level of commitment to serve, consider resigning. Don't sully your reputation by poor attendance and problematic performance. Since healthcare organization boards are composed of the most connected and respected people in town, word quickly gets around regarding directors who pull their weight and those who don't.

MAXIM4
BECOME A PROFESSIONAL DIRECTOR.

Professionals are typically defined as people who engage in occupations full-time for pay, whereas amateurs are those who undertake the same endeavors on a part-time basis without compensation. In this sense, all board members are amateurs. But, the following definitions get closer to the essence of these terms:

- *pro•fes•sion•al* (pra'fêsh-a-nal); A highly committed, knowledgeable, skilled and experienced practitioner.

- *am•a•teur* (am'ã-tur); A person who engages in an activity as a past-time; someone lacking a high level of sophistication and competency.

To make a difference, add value and really govern, boards must be composed of pros. Professional directors, as contrasted to amateurs:

- undertake board service as a vocation - a role that's assumed to perform important tasks; rather than as a hobby, done solely for personal gratification and amusement.

- take their responsibilities seriously; they're not dilettantes.

- are committed to representing community interests; not furthering their own.

- devote considerable time and energy to the job; not just enough to get by.

- are highly knowledgeable, skilled and experienced; not marginal practitioners.

- are actively engaged; not passive.

- are inquisitive and somewhat skeptical; not totally accepting.

- function as checks-and-balances; not "rubber stamps."

- continually increase their competencies; aren't satisfied with their own status quo.

Directorship

- Who are the pros on your board? Who are the amateurs? What differentiates their director practice? Watch the pros and learn from them.

- All groups typically get what they expect and continuously reinforce. To what extent, and how, does your board encourage professional directorship?

- Which aspects of your director practice are professional? Which are amateurish?

M axim 5

KNOW WHAT'S EXPECTED OF YOU.

The price of admission to the best boardrooms is fulfilling (indeed, exceeding) expectations. Be clear about what they are. Vague or totally unrealistic expectations are killers that can sap your motivation, erode the amount/quality of your participation and impair your effectiveness.

Anecdote: I was being interviewed for membership on two nonprofit boards and couldn't accept both appointments. Over dinners with the CEOs and board chairs I asked, "What's expected of me?" Here (paraphrased) are the responses I got: *Chair A*: "Hum, haven't really thought about it. I guess, not too much. We meet every other month for three hours; you'd be expected to serve on several committees and attend our annual retreat." *Chair B*: "This board takes its work very seriously. We feel governance makes a significant difference to our stakeholders and the organization's long-term success. The key is great directors who understand what's expected of them and then deliver. We've thought very carefully about this and have developed a job description. I should have sent you a copy before this interview, but here it is. Look it over and then let's talk."

Directorship

When being interviewed for a board seat, here are some questions you might ask:

• Why am I being considered for appointment to this board? What knowledge, skills, experiences and perspectives are you seeking? What contributions do you think I can make?

• Do you have a director job description or position charter

I can review? [This is a benchmark governance practice. If you'd like to see an illustrative nonprofit healthcare organization *Director Position Charter*, log-on to www.BoardFood.com, go to the navigation aids page and download the document.]

- About how many hours per month or year should I expect to devote as a member of this board?

- What is the term length, and how many terms are members expected to serve before leaving the board?

- When does the board meet (day and time)? How many regularly scheduled meetings are held each year and how long are they? How many special meetings were held last year and how long were they?

- On occasion, can I participate in board meetings telephonically?

- On how many committees will I be required to serve? How often do they meet and for how long? Do I have some input regarding committee assignments?

- Does the board hold annual retreats? Where are they typically held (locally or at a distant location)?

- Am I expected to attend extramural governance educational conferences/seminars? If so, how often?

- What type of organizational events will I be asked to attend during the year?

- Will I be expected (either explicitly or implied) to make personal contributions to the organization? If so, what is the norm? Will I be required to solicit donations from individuals and organizations where I have connections?

Even if not offered, I think it's a must to ask for the opportunity to talk with several current directors. Schedule about an hour with each individually. The key topics should be: the nature of their experiences as directors, both pluses and minuses; and general board climate/culture.

Maxim 6

GET TO KNOW YOUR COLLEAGUES.

Governance is an intensely interpersonal activity. The best boards function as focused, effective, efficient and creative teams. A necessary prerequisite is members who understand one another and where each is coming from. Get to know your fellow directors: their professional/personal histories, perspectives/values, interests, knowledge/skill/experience mix, why they choose to serve and continue serving, and what they want to accomplish.

Although directors need not (and probably shouldn't) be best friends, it's critical they understand and respect one another. Building wholesome and empowering interpersonal relationships takes time and effort. This can't be done through interactions in the boardroom alone; there isn't enough time and it's not a particularly conducive space for doing so.

Anecdote: I once sat on a commercial corporation board where the directors and key executives went on a four-day fishing trip each year to an isolated location. I don't like to fish, and when first told of the annual ritual I thought it was an unnecessary boondoggle. After going on several of them, I came to realize how important they were to our board's healthy/empowering culture and effective teamwork (one of the best I have ever been part of). Members had the opportunity to get into each others' heads and skins. It was time and money well spent.

Directorship

- I've seen boards that don't give any thought or effort to integrating newly appointed directors, other than going around the table and having members briefly introduce themselves. If this is the extent of it, take the "bull by the horns." During the first several months of your service, schedule individual lunch/dinner get-togethers with all other board members. Rest assured, they will be blown away by the gesture and effort. Use the time to build rapport with, and get to know, your colleagues.

- Additionally, if not part of your orientation, insist the CEO arrange meetings for you with each executive team member. Seize the opportunity to learn about them and what they do.

- If your board has someone that provides staff support (i.e., executive assistant, the CEO's secretary, governance coordinator, corporate secretary), take him/her to dinner. More than anyone, he/she will be able to provide you with a feel for the "lay of the land."

- What are some things your board might do to help directors develop better "interpersonal glue" and build the team? It need not be a fishing trip to an isolated location. For some ideas, I suggest you consult: *The Five Dysfunctions of a Team*, by Patrick Lencioni; and *Team Building – Proven Strategies for Improving Team Performance*, by William Dyer, et. al.[1]

---

[1] The full citations for these, and all other books/articles mentioned in the following pages, are provided in the "References and Resources" section.

Maxim 7

If you are a newly appointed director, hook up with a mentor.

A good bit of what goes on in boardrooms is rooted in long chains of events/issues that have evolved over time, linked to a variety of other matters, very subtle, permeated with nuance (i.e., "politics") and complex. Additionally, every board has its own distinctive way of doing business. Your success as a director will depend on how effectively you get up to speed and begin understanding this terrain in terms of boardroom substance and dynamics.

My recommendation: Early in your tenure, enlist an experienced director to serve as your mentor; someone who can help you understand the organization, the board, how it functions and issues coming before it.

Directorship

- If your board doesn't have a formal mentoring program as part of its new director orientation (most don't), talk with the board chair and request that someone is assigned to you to play this role. The individual should be an experienced director (one that's exceptionally competent and high performing) who has the time and skills to work with you for about six months. I recommend the following two books on how to craft a productive mentor-mentee relationship: *The Mentee's Guide to Mentoring*, by Norman Cohen; and *Power Mentoring: How Successful Mentors and Protégés Get the Most Out of Their Relationships*, by Ellen Ensher and Susan Murphy.

- At your first meeting (perhaps during a long conversation over dinner), get an initial "navigational fix." Some things to talk about might include:

  - thumb-nail profiles of each director and key executive,

  - strengths and weakness of the board in terms of how it considers and acts upon issues, plans, proposals and recommendations,

  - the most important boardroom norms; rules-of-the-road (rarely formally codified or even discussed) that guide director behavior and how business is conducted,

  - nature of the board-CEO relationship, and

  - a brief history of how the board has evolved and changed over the last five years or so; particularly seminal events…major successes and failures, how the board coped with them and what was learned.

- Before each board meeting, get on the phone with your mentor and spend some time reviewing the agenda.

  - What are the key issues (both explicit and below the surface)?

  - What is the context and history surrounding items that will be addressed? Why are they on the agenda? What is wanted from the board and how can it make a contribution? What sensitivities (organizational and personal) might emerge?

- After each board meeting, huddle with your mentor to review the meeting and how the board went about its work, in addition to your own performance/contributions.

- If you're an experienced director, offer to mentor a newly appointed one. You'll get far more than you give.

M<small>AXIM</small> 8

I<small>MMEDIATELY</small> <small>BEGIN</small> <small>ACQUIRING</small> <small>AN</small> <small>UNDERSTANDING</small> <small>OF</small> <small>GOVERNANCE</small> <small>AND</small> <small>THE</small> <small>NATURE</small> <small>OF</small> <small>BOARD</small> <small>WORK.</small>

Like other types of work, directorship is a practice grounded on a body of knowledge. You'll pick up some of this in the boardroom over time. But, the underlying and essential fundamentals can't be acquired by repeated observation and practice alone; a little formal learning will be required.

The best "book knowledge" leavens experience. Some things about governance and governing important to understand are:

- the distinctive nature of a nonprofit healthcare organization's stakeholders and how they relate to a board's purpose,

- obligations, responsibilities and roles of nonprofit healthcare organization boards,

- key factors that drive/affect board performance and contributions,

- how boards exercise influence over/in the organizations they govern, and

- the nature of the board–CEO relationship.

I will address these topics, very briefly, in some of the maxims that follow; but, it's a mere "Baskin Robbins taste spoon."

Directorship ⬤━

- To acquire a grounding, I recommend:

  - *Getting to Great: Principles of Health Care Organization Governance*, by Dennis Pointer and James Orlikoff. This book is less than 200 pages, employs a principles format, is chock-full of application sidebars/guides and written in a tight/conversational style. If you want to review the book's table of contents, including a listing of the 72 principles, log-on to www.BoardFood.com, go to the bookshelf page and download the document.

  - *The Excellent Board I* and *The Excellent Board II*, by Karen Gardner (editor), is a compendium of the best articles on a wide variety of governance topics taken from *Trustee Magazine.*

- If you want to move beyond the basics, I suggest: *Governance as Leadership: Reframing the Work of Nonprofit Boards*, by Richard Chait, et. al; and *Boards that Deliver*, by Ram Charan.

Maxim 9
Understand Board Topography.

Nonprofit healthcare organizations are very diverse; accordingly, there's a wide variety of arrangements for governing them. It's important to understand key features of this terrain.

There are two basic *governance structures*: centralized and decentralized.

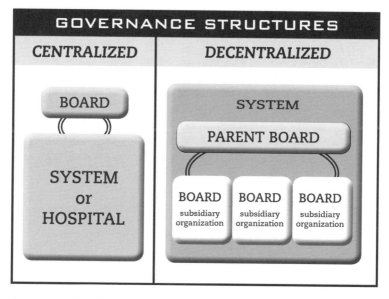

In centralized structures, organizations are governed by a single board. For example, in centralized healthcare systems, subsidiary organizations don't have their own boards. Decentralized systems are composed of a parent and one or more subsidiaries,[2] each of which have boards; governing responsibilities are subdivided and shared among them.

---

[2] Which could include hospitals, long-term care facilities, medical service organization (MSO), medical practices/groups/corporations, a foundation, joint venture corporations, real estate holding company, etc.

There are two different *types of boards*: governing and advisory. Governing boards bear legal fiduciary responsibility and accountability for their organizations. Advisory boards don't ... they provide input, advice and counsel to governing boards and/or management.

There are four primary methods of *director selection*:[3]

- Appointed - One or more directors are chosen by (for example): a stakeholder group such as a sole corporate member (parent board in a health system); or city council for the board of a municipal hospital.

- Elected - Some or all directors are directly elected by (for example): members of the corporation;[4] or the general public in governmental, district hospitals.[5]

- *Ex-officio* - One or more directors are appointed to the board because of other positions they hold. Some illustrations include serving on a board by virtue of being: the CEO; chief/president of the medical staff; president of the volunteer organization or foundation; or holding an elected political office.

- Self-selected - Some or all directors are chosen by presently serving board members.

---

[3] Note: These methods can (and often are) combined in composing a board, for example: Some directors are appointed, some are *ex-officio* and others are self-selected.

[4] Although an increasingly rare governance structure, some nonprofit healthcare organizations have "incorporators," generally individuals meeting minimal criteria who can become members after paying a nominal fee. Typically, their sole function is electing directors nominated by the presently serving board.

[5] District hospitals are supported by public funds; typically, bonds and property taxes. The taxing authorities are established like school districts; voters elect board members who are public officials. States with significant numbers of district hospitals include California, Texas and Washington.

Directorship

- Understand the positioning of your board in this terrain, along the key dimensions:

  - parent/system or subsidiary board,

  - type of board - governing or advisory, and

  - method(s) of director selection - appointed, elected, *ex-officio* and/or self-selected.

- If you serve on the board in a healthcare system that's decentralized: request and review a chart of it's governance structure; and ask to see a document that specifies how governing responsibilities (see *Maxim #16*) are subdivided and coordinated among parent and subsidiary boards (i.e., who does what).

M~AXIM~10
SERVE YOUR APPRENTICESHIP, BUT DO SO QUICKLY.

If you're a newly appointed director, this particular boardroom is foreign territory. You've likely been "plopped down" in an unfamiliar industry/organization, are dealing with issues you don't fully understand and are interacting with other directors who are strangers. You'd be wise to serve an apprenticeship before engaging as a full-fledged journeyman; do so, but do it quickly. Keep in mind, you were appointed to this board because of your knowledge/skills/experience and for the contributions you'll make.

Anecdote: In the early '90s, I joined the board of a NASDAQ listed, healthcare-focused information services company. At my first meeting, I walked into the boardroom and took a seat at the front of the table, to the chair's right. As the meeting progressed I noticed a bit of uneasiness and some sideways glances. At the break I pulled an old friend aside who'd been a director for several years and asked if something was off. He responded: "You sat in John's chair." Mr. _____ was the board's most senior, distinguished and accomplished member. A lesson learned the hard way.

The wise person understands first impressions are critical because they come first and are hard to undo.

Directorship

- What chair you take in the boardroom may be a trivial matter; but what you say or don't, isn't. I recommend sitting back and observing for your first three or four meetings. When you engage, do so by asking questions; not the probing type, but rather those designed to seek information, clarification and elaboration. A person rarely harms oneself by saying too little, at least initially. My greatest embarrassments as a new director have come from making an observation or suggestion when I didn't understand context or know what I was talking about.

- Engage slowly and incrementally over time. Don't come on like "gang busters."

- Recognize that all boards have well-defined authority/ power structures ("pecking orders"). Figure out what they are. Enlist your mentor to help you here (see *Maxim #7*).

- Use your time as an apprentice to: get to know your colleague directors (*Maxim #6*); gain an understanding of healthcare organization governance (*Maxim #8*); and become familiar with the content areas underpinning issues flowing through the boardroom (*Maxim #17*).

Maxim 11

REALIZE GOVERNING IS A DISTINCTIVE ORGANIZATIONAL PRACTICE.

prac•tice (pràk-'tîcë); An activity employing knowledge ("know-what") and skills ("know-how"), sometimes supplemented by technologies, to solve problems and seize opportunities.

Governance, like management and medicine, is a practice; however, when contrasted with them, it's distinctive.

First, governance is part-time and occasional work. While executives, the medical staff and employees are permanent organizational fixtures ... directors are not. Boards convene for short periods of time, they adjourn, and weeks or months pass before they meet again.

Second, due to its part-time nature, board work is episodic and fragmented. It's done in discrete bursts of activity, not continuously. As a consequence, collective memory and momentum is difficult to sustain. No matter how important the issue being addressed, it fades into the background at the end of a meeting and must be • resurrected at the next one.

Third, boards exist only when they meet, between "raps of the gavel."[6] The typical nonprofit healthcare organization board meets for two - three hours, 11 times per year; thus, it has only 22 – 33 hours per year to govern one of society's most important and complex institutions.

Fourth, while management and medicine are individual practices,[7] governance is a "team sport." A director has no

---

[6]   For example, boards, *per se*, don't exist when their committees meet. Committees are board components/sub-groups; they can't (other than in isolated and narrow instances), legally or functionally, discharge full board obligations and responsibilities.

individual authority and power, as governing responsibility rests with the board as a whole.

Directorship

- Many directors, particularly those who practice their professions individually/autonomously (e.g., consultants, physicians, lawyers, accountants), often have difficultly adjusting to a board's collective orientation and collaborative way of doing business. Consensus decision making, after long deliberation and debate, just goes against their grain. How comfortable, experienced and skilled are you at playing the team sport of governance?

- I run across directors who think they can make individual requests of … or even tell … executives, management staff, employees or physicians "what to do." They're missing one of the most fundamental aspects of governance as a collaborative practice.

- Because board attention and work is inherently fragmented … memory, thrust, follow-through and follow-up are often problematic. Systems and procedures must be put in place to increase the seamlessness and continuity of governance work. Your board might consider implementing a follow-up agenda to track all action items for review/assessment at future meetings. Additionally, I recommend that you retain all board/committee meeting agendas and associated back-up materials for one year. This takes a bit of filing cabinet space, but it's helpful as a memory refresher and personal tracking system.

---

[7]   I typically get a push-back on this from conference attendees, board retreat participants and my graduate students; it's always fun to discuss. Clearly, managerial and medical work is supported/facilitated by many people; it couldn't be done without them. However, managerial and clinical decisions are made by individuals. My favorite illustration is to ask a physician whose name is on his/her medical license. It's he or she, not a group.

M<small>AXIM</small>12
RECOGNIZE THE DIFFERENCE BETWEEN GOVERNING AND MANAGING, THEN RESPECT IT.

Management's job is to run the organization; the board's work is to ensure it's run well. The more your board attempts to manage, the less it will govern effectively.

Clearly, the zone between governing and managing is fuzzy. Diligent governing to one director is encroaching on management prerogatives to another. Additionally, the governance-management boundary changes over time. For example: A board might be more directive with a new, relatively inexperienced CEO than with one who's done an outstanding job for years.

General principle: the board's role is to frame issues, question, probe and oversee; management solves problems, seizes opportunities, executes and runs things.

Illustrations help, here's one. A financial problem arises. Days of cash on hand have been falling over the last six months and the organization's liquidity is threatened. The board's job is to: recognize the problem (if it hasn't already been identified and brought to it by management); understand the context and contingencies/constraints; explicitly and precisely convey its expectations (the number of days of cash that should be on hand); hold management accountable for formulating a plan to correct the problem; and then follow-up to ensure management's plan is having the desired effect. The board should not spend time discussing how to solve the problem; this is management's job. Yet, I see boards crossing this governing-management boundary all the time. Such behavior deflect boards from what they should be doing, and wastes a lot of valuable time, while simultaneously disempowering executives.

Here's a metaphor I've found helpful: The board's role is to stay in the balcony, orchestrating and overseeing the dance. Management does the dancing. *Temptations of the director*: Every now and then, directors want to take a spin on the dance floor; it's often more fun than just watching. Put simply: resist it!

An anecdote, my sin: Some years back I was on the board of XYZ Corporation and attending a meeting where the Vice President for Business Development was doing a briefing on a contemplated move into a new and highly competitive market. I started peppering her with recommendations. I've taught graduate-level courses in competitive strategy for the past 25 years and have done extensive consulting in this area with both commercial and healthcare organization clients. Bob, the President/CEO and board chair said: "Denny you're doing it again; crossing the line and dabbling in management. I know you're sinning because I've read your book." Sheepishly, I replied, "You're right; let's move on." Driven by my personal interests and desire to be helpful, I had wandered where I didn't belong. As an aside, this interchange reflects a very healthy boardroom climate: The CEO felt comfortable ushering me back to the balcony.

Directorship

- Pay attention when you begin "drifting down to the dance floor," then pull yourself back. This requires constant vigilance, because the desire to be helpful by sharing your expertise is deeply ingrained. This is particularly true when the issue being discussed is in your professional "sweet spot."

- When a director colleague is approaching, or has crossed, the governance-management boundary, help pull 'em back by providing some feedback; do it lovingly and with humor. Like the "my sin anecdote," healthy boardrooms are characterized by this type of behavior.

- Encourage your board to have a discussion regarding the general principle forwarded in this maxim; whether it should be adopted as a "running rule" and how directors should be reminded of it when they go astray.

Maxim 13

Keep your eyes on the prize.

This maxim is a famous quote from Dr. Martin Luther King, Jr.

Health system boards, hospital boards, medical group boards, home health agency boards, nursing home boards, professional/trade association boards ... quite a diverse lot. But, beyond some superficial differences, they have identical obligations.

The purpose of all nonprofit boards is to represent stakeholders; the rough equivalent of shareholders in commercial corporations. Identifying them can be quite involved; but, a rough first approximation is: stakeholder = the community.[8]

A board's fundamental and overarching obligation is to make sure the organization benefits its stakeholders. Organizations are collections of resources: money, personnel, facilities, equipment, supplies, competencies and capacities. These are means; the end is stakeholder benefit. Boards must ensure that organizational means lead to the end of maximizing stakeholder benefit/value. This is the BIG WHY of governing.

The problem is: In boardrooms, means can overwhelm and eventually displace ends. This dynamic is called *means-ends substitution.*

A board's purpose is to represent the interests of an organization's stakeholders; management's objective is to enhance the organization's performance. A board's purpose and management's objectives are different.

Management's plans, proposals and recommendations are

---

[8]   The community is clearly a nonprofit healthcare organization's primary and ultimate stakeholder. However, this conceptualization is rarely fine-grained enough, as communities are very diverse. Here's a simple illustration: Say you're on the board of a nonprofit condominium homeowners association. Who are the stakeholders? At first glance the answer is easy: those who own units (i.e., equivalent to the community of a nonprofit healthcare organization). Actually, there are probably three stakeholder subgroups: those who own units and live in them, those who own units and rent them out, and those who rent units. Each of these groups has different (and potentially conflicting) needs/interests which the board must represent.

formulated to improve strategic, operational, financial and/or clinical performance. However, when they're being reviewed, discussed, considered and eventually voted on in the boardroom, it's easy for the interests of the organization *per se* to overwhelm and displace those of stakeholders.

Here's the governing challenge: Most often, what's good for the organization also benefits stakeholders. But sometimes it doesn't; what increases organizational performance can decrease stakeholder benefit. It's the board's obligation to be vigilant in such circumstances and carefully assess proposed initiatives from a stakeholder value-added perspective. Management should be concerned about this, but it's the board's responsibility to ensure it.

Anecdote: With the objective of preparing a case study (which never saw the light of day), I interviewed directors serving on the board of a nonprofit health system that was considering the sale of one of its hospitals to a for-profit corporation. Cutting through all of the detail, I found no evidence the board ever seriously assessed the deal's relative costs and benefits from a stakeholder benefit perspective. Management's analysis, contained in a three-inch ring binder, and the board's discussion/deliberation was totally organizational-centric; that is, how the deal would benefit the health system. Put simply: fundamentally flawed governance flowing from a lack of clarity regarding board purpose/obligations and stakeholder interests.

Directorship

- I once sat on a Catholic hospital board where the sister chair (a true saint) began each meeting with a brief reflection/discussion regarding the board's purpose and its obligation to stakeholders. This kept our "eyes on the prize."

- For your board to be truly stakeholder-centric, it must specify the organization's key stakeholders and understand their most important interests. If you'd like to have a *Board Stakeholders Briefing* (which provides much more depth on stakeholders and how to map them, plus numerous non-profit healthcare organization examples), log-on to www.BoardFood.com, go to the <u>navigation aids</u> page and download the document.

- You can learn more about stakeholders by consulting: *Getting to Great: Principles of Health Care Organization Governance* (Chapter 3), by Dennis Pointer and James Orlikoff.

- The foundational/critical importance of stakeholders, as a point of departure for governing, is emphasized in *Building an Exceptional Board: Effective Practices for Health Care Governance – Report of a Blue Ribbon Panel*, published by the Center for Healthcare Governance (CHG), American Hospital Association. You can download a copy, free-of-charge, from www.americangovernance.com, CHG's website.

MAXIM 14

DON'T REPRESENT NARROW INTERESTS OR CONSTITUENCIES.

This is a more nuanced aspect of the preceding maxim.

Consider this, albeit "over-the-top," situation:[9] Friendly Hospital's board is composed of directors who see themselves as representatives of, and advocates for, various special interests. Some illustrations:

- Harry feels it's his duty to represent employees (he's a former union official).

- Gail, president of the medical staff, believes she serves on the board to advance physician interests, especially those of her specialty (radiology).

- Bill is a retired CPA and sings only one note: cost reduction.

- Dan, the only Black on the board, perceives himself as an advocate for the African-American community.

- Sharon has one issue, right-to-life, and isn't interested in anything else.

- Ann sees herself as the standard-bearer for women's issues.

---

[9]   Although embellished, this is a real board for whom I once conducted a retreat. It was a tough two days. None of the members could transcend their own narrow perspectives/interests and consider those of all stakeholders; a crucial starting-point for really governing.

- John, who several years ago made the single largest gift the organization has ever received, is only concerned about insuring his own legacy.

Could this board govern effectively on behalf of all stakeholders? Or would it be torn apart, and eventually rendered impotent, by each director's narrow perspectives and interests?

Your board's job is to represent; but, it must do so by balancing and aligning the different/divergent interests of various stakeholders. What you must not do is serve as a narrowly focused standard-bearer and single-issue advocate.

If your board is composed of members who seek to advance special interests, it will be torn apart by centrifugal forces and its effort to govern fragmented. One director argues on behalf of a particular group; other directors do the same thing from equally narrow perspectives. The board takes on the characteristics of a legislative body or courtroom.

Directorship

- As a director you are a stakeholder agent. Your position is neither a license nor a platform for "beating the drum" regarding issues you hold dear. You have a duty to balance/align the interests of all stakeholders, not representing those of just one or a few.

- *Ex-officio* directors (those who serve on the board by virtue of other positions they hold), face the greatest challenges here.[10] For example, a physician who's a director because he/she is the elected chief of staff. The medical

---

[10]   *Ex-officio* directors have the same obligation as all other board members: to represent stakeholders as a "general class;" that is, balancing/aligning the interests of each stakeholder group, favoring no particular one. Look at it this way: What gets *ex- officio* directors to the boardroom is their membership in a stakeholder group; the board wants/needs the competencies, experiences and perspectives that comes with such membership. However, once in the boardroom *ex-officio* directors breach their fiduciary duty of loyalty (see *Maxim #15*) by solely representing the interests of the groups from which they came.

staff expects this individual to represent their interests. Your board must offer such directors assistance and "air cover:" providing them with gentle reminders when they overstep the boundary; and constantly reminding their physician colleagues they're on the board because of the knowledge, skills, experience and perspectives they bring... not to represent medical staff interests.

M AXIM 15

UNDERSTAND YOUR LEGAL FIDUCIARY DUTIES OF LOYALTY, CARE AND OBEDIENCE IN ADDITION TO DIRECTOR LIABILITIES/PROTECTIONS.

All state nonprofit organization incorporation laws hold that directors have a fiduciary duty to serve as stakeholder agents, acting in ways that protect and advance their interests, carefully and in accordance with the law. You are accountable for being loyal, careful and obedient, and potentially legally liable if you're not.

Loyalty is owed first/primarily to stakeholders and then second/derivatively to the organization. Loyalty to stakeholders always trumps loyalty to the organization. Accordingly, loyalty's center-of-gravity is serving as a stakeholder agent and faithfully representing their interests. You breach this duty when, for example: a material conflict-of-interest influences your decisions; you disclose confidential information that might have a detrimental effect on the organization; you seize a business opportunity for yourself or other parties that legitimately belongs to the organization; you vote for an unlawful distribution of the organization's assets which subverts its charitable purpose and/or results in private inurnment.

Care requires discharging your governing responsibilities with the diligence, prudence and sound judgment equal to that of an ordinarily competent person in similar circumstances. This duty focuses on the process of acting and deciding, not the results. The test is: Was reasonable care exercised? Not: Was the outcome optimal, satisfactory or even tolerable? You are permitted to presume that information, analyses and recommendations provided by others (executives, staff and consultants) are accurate, truthful and informed ... if there are no compelling reasons to believe otherwise. This duty does not require you to be overly cautious, avoiding all risks. Courts are very hesitant to substitute their judgment for those of boards, after the fact. The expectation is simply that directors act carefully, with common sense and informed judgment.

Obedience requires that you obey the law. Directors must avoid acts beyond the board's authority as articulated in applicable laws, court decisions and regulations, in addition to those specified in the organization's own governing documents. To discharge this duty you must: understand the law and the organization's/board's charter, articles of incorporation, bylaws and policies; and abide by them. Unlike the requirement to be careful, the test of fulfilling this duty is not merely good faith intentions, but rather compliance and results. Ignorance is never a justifiable excuse for breaching this duty.

The good news: nonprofit healthcare organization directors are rarely named in lawsuits. The bad news: if you are, it's a hassle. You must be loyal, careful and obedient; if a party feels that you're not, they can sue. In an increasingly litigious society, and given heightened standards of board accountability, such actions are becoming more common. My intent is not to scare you. However, because board membership comes with potential personal liability, it pays to be prudent.

As a director you typically have two protections:[11] indemnification and directors' and officers' (D&O) insurance. Neither is automatic. The first must be provided (typically *via* your board's bylaws), the second has to be purchased by the organization on whose board you serve.

Organizations can choose to indemnify directors (i.e., offer protection against liability and financial loss), although specific provisions vary considerably. If a director is named in a suit arising

---

[11]   In some states there are three: those that have enacted legislation providing the directors of certain charitable nonprofit organizations limited indemnification (or immunity). The provisions of such legislation vary so widely, I've chosen not to discuss them here. My recommendation: ask the organization's counsel for a briefing.

out of board service, he/she may be reimbursed by the organization for expenses incurred (including attorney's fees) and in specified instances for judgments, awards and fines. Typically, expenses are paid by the organization during the action, not after it's resolved. The common standard for such indemnification is: the director acted in good faith and in a manner he/she believed to be in the best interest of the organization and its stakeholders; and (if the action is allegedly criminal), the director had no reasonable cause to believe his/her action was unlawful.

Additionally, an organization may purchase liability insurance that reimburses expenses incurred due to actions for which its directors and officers are covered (e.g., the cost of indemnification); but certain types of claims are typically excluded. D&O insurance covers the organization, not directors directly.

Directorship

- To learn more about your legal fiduciary duties, I recommend: *The Board's Fiduciary Role: Legal Responsibilities of Health Care Governing Boards*, by Fredric Entin, et. al.

Loyalty

- Insist that your board is reminded of, and "re-briefed" by counsel regarding, its duty of loyalty prior to considering, deliberating about and voting on major issues, big deals and large financial transactions.

- With respect to issues coming before your board, acknowledge any potential conflicts-of-interest and seek an opinion regarding their materiality. If the conflict is judged to be material, totally remove yourself from discussing, deliberating, exercising any influence regarding, and voting on, the matter. This is critical to fulfilling your fiduciary duty of loyalty, as material conflicts are among the most common causes of breaching it. See *Maxim #25* where this is addressed in more depth.

- Never talk with outsiders about information/matters deemed to be sensitive or confidential. See *Maxim #26* where this is addressed in more depth.

- Ensure that the independent/external auditor reports to the board any concerns regarding private inurnment arrangements that might jeopardize the organization's charitable purposes and nonprofit status.

Care

- Insist background materials are distributed an adequate amount of time prior to board/committee meetings so directors can carefully review and reflect upon key issues before addressing them.

- Expect analyses prepared by staff and consultants to thoroughly/accurately portray both the positives and negatives of proposed initiatives.

- You must be present and contribute to exercise due care; attend board meetings and participate.

- Come to every board/committee meeting prepared, having carefully read agenda materials and proposals/recommendations up for discussion and vote.

- Always ask for additional information and clarification when you do not understand an issue.

- Insist that adequate time is allocated for questions, elaboration/clarification, discussion, deliberation and debate prior to votes ... especially on important agenda items.

- Prior to votes on important matters, ask for an assessment by counsel regarding whether your board has exercised its duty of care.

- Don't be pressured by apparent overwhelming agreement. In light of the facts, after listening carefully to your director colleagues plus taking a stakeholder perspective, be prepared to vote "no." See *Maxim #31* where this is addressed in more depth.

<u>Obedience</u>

- Request that periodic educational sessions are held on legislative, legal and regulatory developments in addition to their implications for your board.

- Ask for the opinion of legal counsel regarding the applicability of key laws, regulations and court decisions before dealing with important matters and big deals.

- If you've not done so recently, review the organization's articles of incorporation and charter in addition to your board's bylaws.

- Request a book containing all board policies (updated continuously) be provided to you; then periodically review them.

<u>Liabilities and Protections</u>

- These matters are very important, complex and technical. Accordingly, each year, request that the organization's counsel brief your board on potential risks and legal liabilities, in addition to the nature/scope of protections available. If your board's indemnification provisions and D&O insurance coverage haven't been reviewed by an experienced governance/corporate attorney in the last several years, request this be done.

- You might want to have your personal attorney review the board's indemnification policy and D&O insurance. As an extra layer of protection and comfort, ask your attorney for a referral to counsel experienced in governance/corporate law.

- Your best protection against the potential legal liability that comes with board service is to understand your job and do it conscientiously ... and, I might add, heed these 40 maxims!!

M AXIM 16
UNDERSTAND YOUR BOARD'S GOVERNING RESPONSIBILITIES.

The substantive work of governing entails fulfilling responsibilities. The core ones for nonprofit healthcare organization boards are:[12]

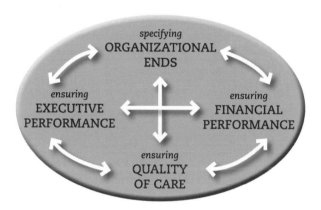

Only the briefest synopsis of these responsibilities are forwarded here as they've been a major focus in four of my previous books.

Ends

Ends are destinations and paths taken. Both are choices, and among the most important organizations make. Formulating/ approving them is a board responsibility.

---

[12]   This model was originally introduced in *Really Governing: How Health System and Hospital Boards Can Make More of a Difference*, by Dennis Pointer and Charles Ewell. It was elaborated and expanded in, *Board Work: Governing Health Care Organizations*, *Getting to Great: Principles of Health Care Organization Governance* and *The High Performance Board: Principles of Nonprofit Organization Governance*, all by Dennis Pointer and James Orlikoff. The model has become a standard framework for describing/prescribing the responsibilities of nonprofit healthcare organization boards. See, for example: *Building an Exceptional Board*, Report of a Blue Ribbon Panel on Health Care Governance (Center for Healthcare Governance, American Hospital Association); and *Board Roles and Responsibilities: Elements of Governance* (The Governance Institute).

In attending to ends, your board defines the organization: what it is and isn't; what it will and will not become. Governance begins here. Other responsibilities (for executive performance, quality of care and financial performance) all flow from this one. To fulfill this responsibility, your board must:

- provide input regarding, and assist in formulating/approving the organization's vision,[13]

- review/approve key organization-wide goals,[14]

- ensure management strategies[15] are aligned with the vision and key goals, and

- monitor/assess how well the vision is being fulfilled, key goals are accomplished and strategies are being pursued, in addition to expecting corrective action if problems are detected.

Executive Performance

A board has one direct report, the CEO; he/she is its agent and delegated authority to manage the organization's affairs.

The board-CEO relationship is intricate and complex because the CEO: is simultaneously the board's "subordinate" (hired and fired by it) and a colleague director (in over 80 percent of health systems and hospitals); and exerts a significant influence over the

---

[13] Highly successful organizations share one thing in common: they have distinctive, explicit, precise, fine-grained and empowering visions. The reason is simple: an organization cannot achieve that which its leadership is unable to envision. Visions spell the difference between purposefully moving into the future versus aimlessly wandering there. A vision specifies what an organization should/must become in order to maximize stakeholder benefit. The best way to formulate and codify a vision is not a prose statement, but rather a list of specific characteristics regarding what the organization should look like, at its very best, in the future.

[14] Goals are the most important things an organization must accomplish for its vision to be fulfilled; they increase a vision's specificity and "density."

[15] Strategies are specific plans for deploying an organization's resources (fiscal, human, facilities, equipment, supplies, etc.) to achieve key goals.

42

amount/type of information the board receives and its agenda.

Your board is responsible and accountable for the CEO's performance; it must:

- recruit and select the CEO,

- assess the CEO's performance,

- adjust the CEO's compensation, and

- should the need arise, terminate the CEO's employment relationship with the organization.

Quality of Care

The responsibility for ensuring quality care is unique to boards of organizations that provide healthcare services.[16] Other nonprofit organization and commercial corporation boards can delegate this to management.

Healthcare quality is multi-dimensional and encompasses clinical quality, patient safety and customer-patient/guest satisfaction. This aspect of governing typically causes directors their greatest trepidations because: of the complexity and mystique of medical work; and most, lacking clinical expertise, find it unreasonable to be asked to assume responsibility for processes they'll never fully comprehend.

To fulfill this responsibility, your board must:

- formulate/approve organization-wide quality objectives,

- credential the medical staff (appoint/reappoint practitioners and specify their privileges),

---

[16]   Healthcare organizations, *via* the authority vested in their boards, bear ultimate responsibility and accountability for the quality of care due to a long series of court decisions, Federal legislation, regulatory mandates and accreditation requirements.

- ensure that necessary quality, utilization and risk management systems are in place and functioning effectively, and

- monitor/assess the quality of care provided and expect corrective action if problems are detected.

Financial Performance

Nonprofit healthcare organizations are simultaneously community benefit institutions and business entities. As the latter, they must: accumulate and productively deploy fiscal resources; engage in value-added economic transactions; and produce positive margins, as nonprofit doesn't mean no-profit.

Your board is responsible and accountable for the organization's financial performance and condition; it must:

- formulate/approve organization-wide financial objectives,

- ensure financial/capital plans are aligned with, and will likely accomplish, financial objectives,

- monitor/assess financial performance/condition and expect corrective action if problems are detected,

- ensure the organization's credit worthiness,

- ensure necessary internal controls are in place, and

- oversee the independent/external audit and ensure financial statements fully/fairly reflect the organization's financial condition.

Responsibilities Overall

These four core responsibilities are grounded on, and flow from, board legal fiduciary duties (see *Maxim #15*). That is, for your board to be both loyal (to stakeholders, representing their interests) and careful (overseeing the organization's affairs), it must attend to ends, executive performance, quality of care and finances. There are other things your board might *choose* to do, but fulfilling these responsibilities are things your board *must* do.

Focus

Anecdote: When conducting retreats I often ask directors to take out a sheet of paper and write down the most important responsibilities of healthcare organization boards; the key things they must do, their critical functions. The responses are always quite varied. Although there's occasional overlap on a few individual items, there's never general agreement about the basics.[17] Richard thinks boards should be doing A, B, C and D; Mary thinks it should be B, D, H, J and R; Dan feels the most important responsibilities are B, H, P, U and W; Jane isn't sure and Glen hasn't given it much thought.

Peter Drucker defines effectiveness as "doing the right things" (in contrast to efficiency which is "doing things right"). Your board cannot be effective unless there's agreement among directors regarding the right things they must do. Without this your board will: not have a coherent framework for allocating its most precious resource of director attention; lack focus; waste time, energy and effort; and drift toward peripheral and tangential issues ... increasingly, sheer activity replaces productive work.

Laser-like focus on responsibilities is essential for a board to be effective. Not only does this define what your board should be doing; but equally, if not more important, specifies what it shouldn't. Willie Nelson (one of my favorite philosophers) says: "If the next pot of chili taste better than the last, it's probably due to what's left out, not what's been added."

---

[17] I've conducted this exercise hundreds of times, always with similar outcomes. If you doubt the results, or would just like to replicate the experiment, try it at your next board meeting.

- It's critical that directors have a shared and explicit/precise definition of your board's core responsibilities: the substance of governance work. Achieving this will require some time and effort. A few suggestions:

  - Circulate readings regarding the core board responsibility model to directors, taken from *Board Work* (Chapter 4) and *Getting to Great: Principles of Healthcare Organization Governance* (Chapter 4).

  - Discuss this model at a special board meeting or retreat. See if it makes sense and explore its implications (e.g., board meeting agenda planning and management and committee structure).

- If you'd like to see an illustrative *Board Charter* crafted in-line with this responsibility model, log-on to www.BoardFood.com, go to the navigation aids page and download the document.

Maxim 17

Acquire an increasingly sophisticated understanding of content areas underpinning issues your board will be addressing.

Being a great director demands solid general intelligence, common sense, good business judgment, well-rounded experience and a splash of wisdom. However, governance is not a competence-free zone; it requires knowledge in areas grounding/framing issues with which your board will be dealing. Among the most important are:

- the structure and functioning of the U.S. healthcare industry,

- factors that affect/drive a healthcare organization's strategic and competitive advantage,

- factors that affect/drive a healthcare organization's operational effectiveness and efficiency,

- factors that affect/drive healthcare quality (including clinical quality, patient safety and service quality),

- the nature/challenges of contemporary medical practice and different physician – healthcare organization relationship options, and

- factors that affect/drive a healthcare organization's financial performance and condition.

You don't need to master all this immediately. But, let there be no doubt about it, your success as a director will ultimately depend on how well you understand this stuff.

Directorship

- Work with the board chair and/or CEO to design a cus-tom-crafted development plan to begin acquiring these competencies. A reading program can be a good way to start. Here are some of my top picks:

  - The Healthcare Industry - *The U.S. Health Care Industry: A Primer for Board Members*, by Dennis Pointer and Stephen Williams; and *The U.S. Health Care Delivery System: Fundamental Facts, Definitions and Statistics*, by Sara Beazley, et. al. [if you'd like to review the table of contents for *The U.S. Health Care Industry: A Primer for Board Members*, log-on to www.BoardFood.com, go to the book-shelf page and download the document.]

  - Healthcare Organization Markets and Strategic/Com-petitive Fitness - *Health Care Strategy for Uncertain Times*, by Marion Jennings (editor).

  - Healthcare Organization Operating Fitness - *The Well-Managed Health Care Organization*, by John Griffith and Ken White. [This is a textbook for graduate students in health administration and not a light read. But, in one volume, every facet of a hospital's operation is covered; it's a great overview and reference.]

  - Quality of Care - *The Quality Advantage*, by Julianne Morath; *10 Powerful Ideas for Improving Patient Care*, by James Reinertsen and Wim Schellekens; and *If Disney Ran Your Hospital: 9½ Things You Would Do Differently*, by Fred Lee.

- Physicians and Contemporary Medical Practice - *Learning to Play God*, by Robert Marion; *The Next Generation of Physician–Health System Partnerships*, by Craig Holm; and "How to Improve Hospital-Physician Relationships," in *Frontiers of Health Services Management*, by Joe Bujak.

- Financial Fitness - *Best Practice Financial Management: Six Key Concepts for Healthcare Leaders*, by Kenneth Kaufman.

- If you'd like to have a copy of *The Essential Governing Bibliography*, log-on to www.BoardFood.com, go to the bookshelf page and download the document.

• One of the easiest (and most fun) ways to develop your governing competencies is to attend educational events designed specifically for healthcare organization directors. There are several options:

- Many state hospital associations include sessions for directors on a wide variety of topics at their annual meetings. Make it a point to ask your CEO to be kept informed of these programs.

- Several organizations specialize in providing board development and director education. Among the best are: Center for Healthcare Governance, American Hospital Association (www.americangovernance.com); the Estes Park Institute (www.estespark.org); and the Governance Institute (www.governanceinstitute.com). Each offers three-four day conferences multiple times throughout the year at a variety of locations across the country. Most of the content areas noted previously are covered in their curricula. They feature first-rate presenters, and you'll have the opportunity to interact with directors from other organizations. Ask your board chair and CEO about attending. I've found the greatest benefit occurs when a group of directors, in addition to the CEO (and/or another executive team member), attend together.

- The Institute for Healthcare Improvement (www.ihi.org) is, in my judgment, the nation's premier organization dedicated to enhancing clinical quality and patient safety. They conduct an Annual National Forum on Quality Improvement in Healthcare (which, drawing over 6,000 attendees, is now the largest professional meeting in the industry); a five-day healthcare quality improvement workshop for teams of healthcare organization directors, executives and physician leaders; and a two-day conference, "From the Top: The Role of the Board in Quality and Safety." Their website is the go-to location for high quality (and free) resources: white papers, monographs, articles, guides, video clips and annotated bibliographies.

Maxim 18

Develop (or enhance) your healthcare organization-specific financial literacy.

Bluntly stated: It's impossible to be a good, let alone a *great*, healthcare organization director without possessing basic financial literacy. The areas of accounting and finance[18] provide the means for: recording all sorts of (but not all) activity taking place in an organization; quantifying transactions, both internal and between the organization and external entities; depicting an organization's financial status/condition; and planning for the future.

Healthcare organizations are social institutions; critical components of their community's infrastructure. Simultaneously, they are large and complex economic entities whose financial activity exceeds hundreds of millions, and often billions, of dollars. Accounting/finance is the "language of business." Without fluency in this language, directors are rendered sightless, hearing impaired and speechless in the boardroom.

Your board will want to have a few members who are accounting/finance pros, but all directors must possess basic literacy. If you are a financial neophyte, you'll need to build some competencies from scratch. If you've taken undergraduate or graduate courses in this stuff or had some practical experience in other sectors, you'll need to acquaint yourself with the distinctive aspects of healthcare accounting and finance.

---

[18] The discipline of accounting records economic transactions and summarizes them in financial statements; it focuses on an organization's past. The discipline of financial management uses accounting information to analyze and plan; it focuses on an organization's future.

You must:

- understand factors that affect/drive a healthcare organization's financial performance and condition (addressed in *Maxim #17*),

- be able to read, analyze and interpret the organization's basic financial documents, including the revenue/expense statement, balance sheet and statement of cash flows,

- understand the basics of financial planning and be able to participate in reviewing/approving the organization's annual financial plan,

- understand the basics of capital planning and be able to participate in reviewing/approving the organization's capital plan in addition to specific projects,

- be able to participate in monitoring and assessing the organization's financial performance/condition,

- understand factors affecting the organization's credit worthiness,

- understand the internal audit function and be able to participate in ensuring appropriate controls are in place, and

- understand, and be able to participate in, ensuring the organization's financial integrity/credibility through the annual independent audit.

All of these competencies are absolutely essential to fulfilling your fiduciary duty of care (*see Maxim #15*).

I estimate that less than 50 percent of the typical community hospital's board members possess basic financial literacy (the knowledge and skills noted above). It's higher for boards of healthcare systems. Unquestionably, this significantly impairs governing performance and contributions.

One way to solve the problem is to recruit only directors who are financially literate, and some governance pundits have suggested doing so. In my judgment, this bad idea dramatically reduces the overall experience, skill and perspective diversity of healthcare organization boards. Better to recruit broadly and then develop the financial competencies of directors early in their term of service. The "fly in the ointment" is that most boards don't have well designed and executed director-focused financial development programs in place.

Directorship

- The first, and essential, step to developing a competency is recognizing that a deficiency exists. Review the list of knowledge/skills above and do an honest assessment of yourself. How do you stack up? What are your areas of strength and weakness?

- For a good start and overview, I recommend *Essentials of Health Care Organization Finance: A Primer for Board Members*, by Dennis Pointer and Dennis Stillman. This is a collaborative effort between a governance guy (me) and an accounting/finance pro (Stillman is a faculty colleague of mine at UW, was the chief financial officer at University of Washington Medical Center, is a CPA and Fellow of the Healthcare Financial Management Association). We wrote this because there was no director-friendly and governance-focused finance book available. It's less than 180 pages, covers all the basics and no previous accounting/finance knowledge is assumed. If you'd like to review the table of contents for this book, log-on to www.BoardFood.com, go to the bookshelf page and download the document.

- As you read *Essentials,* consider meeting with the chief financial officer (or someone else in the finance department that can transcend "CPA-speak") and do a few tutorials, applying the concepts addressed in the book to your organization's financial statements. Perhaps, there are a few other directors who'd like to join you for such sessions.

- Suggest that some finance-focused, in-service educational programs be conducted for your board. If folks in the finance department have neither the inclination nor teaching skills to undertake this, check with the accounting firm who does the organization's independent audit.

- Often, the type of financial information presented to boards is pulled directly from the organization's management information system. This stuff provides executives (all of whom are financially savvy) what they require to manage the organization, but it's generally not what directors need to govern. Suggest that all key financial documents presented to your board (e.g., revenue/expense statement, balance sheet, statement of cash flows, operating statistics, annual budget, annual financial plan, annual capital plan and capital proposals) be customized for it, in terms of format/form and level of detail. *Essentials* has numerous illustrations of how this should be done. The point is an important one: Often directors, who are non-financial pros, have trouble understanding and interpreting the organization's financial documents ... not due to their lack of basic financial literacy, but because they aren't designed/prepared for consumption by directors; they're just not board-friendly.

  - If something isn't clear, always ask. Chances are, you're not alone.

M AXIM 19

IF YOU'RE THE BOARD CHAIR, LEARN HOW TO RUN EFFECTIVE AND EFFICIENT MEETINGS.

Governance work gets done at meetings. How, and how well, they're planned and conducted has a huge impact on a board's performance/contributions.

One of the most important determinants of a meeting's effectiveness/efficiency is chair knowledge/skills in the areas of agenda planning and process facilitation. This is not acquired naturally or by just chairing meetings repeatedly. Practice alone doesn't make perfect.

Directorship

- Here's some great books:

  - *First Aid for Meetings*, by Charlie Hawkins,

  - *Meetings That Work! A Practical Guide to Shorter and More Productive Meetings*, by Richard Chang and Kevin Kehoe,

  - *How to Conduct Productive Meetings*, by Donald Kirkpatrick, and

  - *Meeting Excellence: 33 Tools to Lead Meetings that Get Results*, by Glen Parker and Robert Hoffman.

- Most universities and colleges offer courses/programs on meeting design, management and facilitation. Check them out. This can be an effective, efficient and low cost way to develop essential skills.

- When combined with either or both of the above, the best way to improve your chair skills is through coaching. Get the organization to retain someone with the necessary expertise and experience (e.g., university faculty member or consultant). Have them observe board meetings (usually six-eight sessions are needed) and, at the conclusion of each, sit with you for about an hour to analyze/assess the meeting ("replay the game films") and offer advice regarding how it might have been designed/managed/facilitated differently and better.

- I recommend allocating 15 minutes at the end of every board meeting for reflection, evaluation and performance improvement action planning. Questions that might be asked and discussed are:

  - How well prepared and "on target" were the meeting's preparatory materials? What should be done to improve them?

  - What percentage of meeting time was spent just listening to briefings, reports and background presentations? What proportion of this was really necessary? Are there alternative ways to convey this information?

  - How much time was spent dealing with relatively low-leverage, peripheral matters/issues? What were they? What could be done to reduce this in the future?

  - How equal was director participation? What might be done to even it out?

  - Overall, to what extent was this meeting an effective/ efficient use of our valuable time?

- Ask each director to respond: "If I could change just one thing about this meeting to improve its effectiveness/efficiency/creativity, it would be _____."

- Ask each director to respond: "To improve this meeting, I should have _____."

- Ask each director to respond: "To enhance meeting effectiveness/efficiency, the chair should consider altering his/her style of facilitation by _____." [If this is deemed too threatening to discuss openly, each director might write his/her recommendation on a piece of paper.]

- Expect some initial resistance. The first half-dozen meetings where this is undertaken, will be uncomfortable and not very productive (as it takes time to build the trust required for candor and specificity). But, with perseverance, it will bear valuable fruit.

• If you'd like to have a *Board Meeting Quick-Assessment Form*, log-on to www.BoardFood.com, go to the navigation aids page and download the document.

MAXIM 20

DO YOUR HOMEWORK.

Come to meetings prepared, fully understanding agenda items and ready to discuss, deliberate and vote on them. I recommend three activities:

- First, crack the agenda book and skim through all of it. Get a general feel for what's likely to be the meeting's ebb and flow.

- Second, go back and carefully read/digest material dealing with the key agenda items; those that will be actively discussed by your board and/or voted on. I do this with a hi-lighter in hand.

- Third, make marginal notes capturing your observations and questions. Plan on spending some serious time preparing for the meeting in order to effectively participate in it; this is a necessary and valuable investment.

Directorship

- Many times directors don't thoroughly read and digest board meeting background materials because they're too voluminous, poorly prepared/organized and arrive late. Expect the agenda books for your board to be:

  - professionally designed, prepared and written,

  - parsimonious - providing the minimum necessary amount of information you need to understand and weigh-in on an issue … I like one-page summaries prepared for all key agenda items, and

- delivered an adequate amount of time before the meeting ... I recommend about one week (early enough that you have time to attend to it, not so early that it gets "misplaced" at the bottom of your inbox).

• After reading through the agenda book, if you have any questions or reservations regarding an item, consider raising them with the board chair before the meeting. Sometimes all it takes is a brief phone conversation. Several things are accomplished: first, you get additional information and/or clarification; second, the chair is provided with a heads-up about your concern; and third, this avoids throwing a "hand grenade" during the meeting.

MAXIM 21

SHOW UP.

The prerequisite of faithful/effective directorship is attending board and committee meetings. You can attend and contribute little; but it's impossible to contribute if you're not at the table. Actions always speak louder than words. Your absence says to colleagues that other commitments are more important and it robs the board of your contributions. Additionally, you are accountable (and potentially liable) for actions undertaken when you're not present.

Absenteeism is a significant problem that saps board strength and diminishes effectiveness, efficiency and creativity. Surveys indicate that approximately 20 percent of directors are absent from regularly scheduled board meetings. Given the typical healthcare organization board has 15 members, that's three people every meeting. The big problem: it's never the same folks. Recall that governance is a team sport. With rotating absenteeism, the team's composition is always changing. This makes it difficult to maintain focus and momentum. First, either extra time is required (at every meeting) to bring those who were AWOL up to speed, or the board moves ahead without everyone in the same place. Second, the board's collective memory is compromised because, no matter how good the review of what transpired at a past meeting, completeness/detail/nuance is inevitably lost.

Directorship

- Most boards schedule their meetings on a set day of the month and specific time (e.g., the third Tuesday at 7:00 PM). Once your board's meeting schedule is set for the year, enter it into your calendar, PDA or whatever ... immediately, then hold these dates sacrosanct.

- I presently sit on a board, which convenes four times per year for 1.5 days per meeting. No excused absences are granted, with the exception of dire personal emergencies. Missing a meeting is a tripwire for a serious conversation with the president/CEO/chair. Miss two meetings during the year and you're on your way out. This is just one of many ways the board reinforces its expectation of professional directorship (see *Maxim #4*).

- Boards want to attract the very best people. But these folks are very busy and have a host of other commitments (typically business travel). This is a "catch-22" and dilemma. One partial work-around is to make it easier for directors to occasionally participate in board meetings at-a-distance. Several things are required:

  - First, the bylaws may have to be amended to allow telephone conference participation equivalent to physical presence.

  - Second, an investment will need to be made in state-of-the-art telephone conferencing equipment in the boardroom (not stuff bought at the local discount electronics store).

  - Third, to really do it right, PowerPoint™ presentations and other materials displayed in the boardroom will need to be video-streamed in real time *via* the internet to directors on their laptop PCs in distant locations. There are a number of companies that provide these services. See for example: gotomeetings.com and gatherplace.net.

Maxim 22

PARTICIPATE.

Don't be a spectator. Contribute your knowledge, skills, experience and perspectives ... and above all, wisdom ... regarding matters coming before your board. Effective participation requires four real-time activities:

- *understanding* issues, plans, proposals and recommendations forwarded to your board,

- *listening* to the views of colleague directors, fully comprehending what they are saying,

- *thinking/reflecting* - processing information and juxtaposing/integrating it with what you already know, think and believe, and

- *talking* - sharing your ideas and opinions articulately (simply, clearly, crisply) so they're easily understood.

The best boardrooms are characterized by vigorous discussion, delibertion and debate; engaged, active, energetic and thoughtful participation.

Anecdote: My office at the University of Washington overlooks the channel between Lake Union and Lake Washington. Early in the morning, UW skull crews are out practicing. Everyone has their hands on the oars and are rowing hard. Winning skull crews have a lot in common with winning boards when it comes to participation.

- Great boards spend most of their meeting time talking, not passively listening to background briefings plus updates and reports from management, the medical staff and their own committees. Could your board really govern if it spent 100 percent of its time just listening? Of course not! What's your board's relative percentage of listening to talking? If listening exceeds 50 percent (and for most boards it does), the limited amount of active, engaged participation is problematic.

- Suggest your board try video or audio taping some briefing/background reports and sending them out with the agenda book. The CEO's board update might be a place to start. In the meeting, with all directors having viewed/listened to the tape, valuable face-to-face time can then be devoted to Q&A and discussion of the content. If it works, this can be extended to board committee reports. Think of the amount of precious boardroom time that will be made available for discussion rather than just listening.

- Director participation should be roughly equal. No one dominates the discussion, nobody checks-out. How characteristic is this of your board?

- Don't grandstand, talking just to flex your cerebral muscle. This turns off your colleagues, wastes precious meeting time and deflects the board's attention.

- Be one who draws out, and encourages, other members' participation.

- Fabricate and share half-baked ideas. Fully-baked ones are tightly structured, fleshed-out and complete; typically, they can only be accepted or rejected pretty much as-is. Half-baked ideas are a mosaic of ingredients that can be rearranged, tossed out or added to; they're ready-made for modification by others' contributions. Group process research shows that creativity is increased as more half-baked ideas are forwarded.

- If you have the inclination and talent (and it takes a lot), play the role of summarizer. The best boardroom deliberations unfold at a blistering pace; ideas, facts, opinions and questions abound. It's helpful to have someone review the discussion: the sequence of what's been said, how ideas are related to one another (or don't) and what has been left out. Groups need short-term memories and maps.

- Demand deliberative patience. Especially for big issues, ensure everyone has a chance to ask questions, express concerns and say their piece. Silence is typically not the best gauge that things have been fully discussed. It's best to ask those who have not said anything to weigh-in: "_____, you've been quiet. What do you think about this? I respect your opinion and would love to hear from you."

M AXIM 23

QUESTION.

One of your most important director tasks is to ask questions. A flurry of plans, proposals and recommendations fly through the boardroom; from management, the medical staff and board committees. Your board's job is to vet them.

> *vet•ting* (vet'-îng); Subjecting something to thorough/careful examination and scrutiny in order to ensure its soundness.

Issue/initiative vetting is done by asking probing questions; here are some good general ones:

- Why is this on the agenda? Why does it warrant our attention?

- What are the desired/anticipated outcomes - strategically, financially, operationally, clinically?

- From a stakeholder perspective, what are the anticipated benefits and potential liabilities?

- What are the most critical assumptions and estimates on which this is based? How were they made and tested?

- What other alternatives were considered? Why were they rejected?

- What are the most likely things that could go wrong? What might be their consequences?

- What implementation planning has been undertaken? What are the most significant execution challenges?

Directorship

- There's an inverse square law of governance: The amount of time a board spends discussing and deliberating an issue is often inversely proportional to its complexity + importance. Why? Simple and less consequential things are easy to understand and analyze.

- Don't be timid. When your gut tells you that things aren't well thought-out, probe until your reservations are resolved.

- Don't be put off by smoke and B.S.; ill-conceived proposals are usually blanketed and riddled with it.

- The ability to ask on-point, probing questions is one of the most important skills of a great director. I strongly recommend: *The 7 Powers of Questions*, by Dorothy Leads; *Leading with Questions*, by Michael Marquardt; and *Making Questions Work*, by Dorothy Srachan.

MAXIM 24
PLAY DEVIL'S ADVOCATE.

Two separate teams are appointed by the Vatican Curia when preparing a proposal for the Pope to beatify or canonize someone: a proselytizer, who makes the positive argument, and a devil's advocate, who argues against it.

As a governing tool, a devil's advocate makes the contrary case ... not necessarily because he/she is opposed to the initiative, but to ensure: complete exploration and thorough analysis; full investigation of alternatives; deliberative reflection; and consideration of potential negative consequences/impacts. It's the ultimate check-and-balance mechanism that ensures a board is fulfilling its duty of care (see *Maxim #15*).

Plans, proposals and recommendations requiring board discussion/action come fully staffed-out: well prepared, complete, weighty, lots of supporting data with arguments persuasively constructed and ready to be approved. It's management's job to proselytize. Your board's role is to be a bit skeptical (but not paranoid); challenging, questioning, fleshing-out and analyzing what's being proposed.

An editorial opinion: I'm convinced that most major organizational debacles that have received above-the-fold coverage in the press (of which Enron and AHERF were the "poster children")[19] could have been avoided by institutionalized board devil's advocacy. It is an absolutely essential characteristic of empowered and effective boardrooms. Recent governance history teaches us that boards must be far tougher and more skeptical

---

[19]   Enron and AHERF (Allegheny Health Education and Research Foundation, a health system that operated in the Pittsburg and Philadelphia markets) are the largest U.S. commercial corporation and nonprofit organization bankruptcies in history. The role of governance in these organizations' demise has been the subject of much study; see, for example, *The Role of the Board of Directors in Enron's Collapse* (Permanent Subcommittee on Investigations, US Senate); and "The Fall of the House of AHERF" (*Health Affairs*), by Lawton Burns, et. al. If you want a copy of the Senate report on Enron, log-on to www.BoardFood.com, go to the other resources page and download the document.

than they've been in the past.

Directorship

- Every director should, occasionally, play the role of devil's advocate. This is an extension of your responsibility to question (*Maxim #23*). Recognize this is lonely and always difficult to do; it's far easier to go with the flow.

- Your board will be occasionally faced with really big deals such as a: merger or acquisition; disposition of a major asset; significant alteration in course (vision and strategy); bond financing and large capital investment decisions. In such cases, suggest the board appoint several directors to function as a formal devil's advocate team. They must be provided with the time, resources, staff assistance and (possibly) consulting support to perform their role well. Then, their contrary case must be heard and entertained by your board.

MAXIM 25

ACKNOWLEDGE CONFLICTS-OF-INTERESTS AND TOTALLY DISENGAGE WHEN YOU HAVE ONE.

Because of the fiduciary duty of loyalty (*Maxim #15*), you're expected to act in the best interest of the organization plus its stakeholders and, accordingly, are prohibited from using your membership on the board for personal gain or the benefit of others. In order to potentially influence your judgment, a conflict must be material (i.e., important, not inconsequential or peripheral). Recognize that existence of a material conflict *per se*, not whether it actually affects your decision, is what's important. There are two types of conflicts: general and limited.

General conflicts are so pervasive and consequential that they compromise your ability to serve as a director who faithfully represents organization/stakeholder interests. For example, you are a nonprofit healthcare organization director and simultaneously a:

- board member of a like-type competitor organization,

- principal (director or senior executive) in the firm that's the organization's investment or commercial banker,

- partner in a law firm that does all of the organization's extramural legal work, or

- executive or director of a health plan that has major contracts with the organization.

Limited conflicts are those that could affect your judgment regarding specific issues coming before the board. For example, you're a director and simultaneously a:

- executive, director or major shareholder/owner of a firm that is bidding on a contract to install a new computerized clinical information system in the organization,

- spouse of the CEO of a firm that has a large outsourcing contract, or

- physician who is an owner/partner of an enterprise (e.g., ambulatory surgical facility, reference laboratory) that competes with the organization in a specific line of business.

Ponder this: Would you want your board composed entirely of individuals who have no potential limited conflicts-of-interests? If you think about it for a moment, I think your answer is "no." If so, directors would neither be connected to, nor involved with, other important organizations/institutions. Your board wants directors with limited (not general) conflicts; but it must have a way of ensuring such conflicts don't materially influence board decision making.

Directorship

- General conflicts-of-interest are so pervasive that, if you have one, you should not accept appointment to the board, or, if already serving, tender your resignation. Before doing so, consult with the organization's counsel and your own attorney to make sure that a conflict really exists. If it does, and you accept a board appointment or continue as a director, you put the organization and yourself in potential jeopardy.

- When a limited conflict-of-interest arises, you should request an opinion from the chair or full board regarding whether it's material. If judged to be so, you should not participate in any board dealings regarding the matter. This includes discussions with executives and other directors, participation in board or committee meetings (you should leave the room), and board vote. Note: the recommendation is total withdrawal, not just abstaining from the vote.

- Prior to board discussion and deliberation regarding really big deals, someone should ask: "Does anyone have a potential material conflict-of-interest?"

- Given the present climate of accountability and transparency, it's prudent to have a board conflict-of-interest policy and associated guidelines/attestation for directors to list (at the time of initial appointment and renewal of term) potential material conflicts-of-interest. If you'd like to see an illustrative *Conflict-of-Interest Protocol*, log-on to www.BoardFood.com, go to the navigation aids page and download the document.

- Legal counsel should brief your board on conflict-of-interest issues and director requirements annually.

MAXIM 26

KEEP SENSITIVE INFORMATION CONFIDENTIAL.

As a director you will be privy to confidential information, defined as: that, which if shared with outsiders, could potentially jeopardize the organization's ability to act in the best interests of its stakeholders. This includes data, ideas, analyses, opinions, plans and decisions, whether communicated to you in documents or verbally. Your fiduciary duties of loyalty and care (see *Maxim #15*) requires you keep such information confidential, not sharing it with any unauthorized persons/groups, either intentionally or accidentally. This duty is in-force not only during your tenure, but also after you leave the board.

Things that might be considered confidential include, but are not limited to, information about:

- certain medical staff credentialing and disciplinary action support materials,

- CEO and executive team performance evaluations,

- risk management and pending malpractice claims/litigation,

- market and competitors analyses,

- strategic, financial and capital plans,

- contract terms for the provision of services (with health plans and insurance companies),

- analyses/recommendations regarding pending mergers, acquisitions and disposition of major assets,

- analyses/recommendations regarding pending land and facilities purchases,

- contracts with major vendors, and/or

- contracts with physicians and medical groups.

Directorship

- It's both prudent (from the organization's perspective) and helpful (for you) to have a formal confidentiality agreement signed by directors upon initial appointment and renewal of term. This agreement should spell-out the expectation of confidentiality plus its importance to the organization and stakeholders; a general definition, and illustration, of the types of information/materials deemed to be sensitive; and the need for confidentiality in addition to its relationship to a director's legal fiduciary duty of loyalty and care. If you'd like to see an illustrative *Director Confidentiality Agreement*, log-on to www.BoardFood.com, go to the navigational aids page and download the document.

- The biggest challenge for directors is generally not poor intentions (most want to do the right thing), but not knowing what type of information is confidential. Accordingly, I recommend:

  - formally going into "confidential sessions" when sensitive matters are being discussed and specifically noting the reasons for doing so, and

- marking all board materials, whether in the agenda book or distributed during a meeting, that are confidential.

• If you have any questions about what information and materials should be treated as confidential, always ask and seek clarification.

• Legal counsel should brief your board on confidentiality issues and director requirements annually.

MAXIM 27
BE ETHICAL.

The ethical aspects of governing have been accorded little attention in the scholarly and professional literature, but they've gotten "above the fold" coverage in the popular press.

Directors have a legal duty to be careful and abide by the law, but there are no requirements to behave ethically. However, to fulfill their responsibilities on behalf of stakeholders, directors' decisions and actions must be grounded on and driven by ethical considerations, particularly in nonprofit healthcare organizations.

A lot of ink has been spilled on the topic of ethics, and even the briefest treatment is beyond the scope of this book. The discipline deals with what is "good" (as contrasted to what's legal and/or prudent). *Good* is defined, and principles for achieving it formulated. Ethical principles are based on rules of logic and differ from morals and norms.[20] Most of what's been written is pretty dense and not composed in lucid prose; but when distilled, it's very helpful.

Ethical directorship is about having good intentions, behaving in good ways, achieving good outcomes, and deliberately/consciously employing some time-tested principles as guides for making decisions and acting.

The *Ethical Pyramid* is a model many boards have found helpful for increasing their governing quality:[21]

---

[20] Morals and norms also deal with what is good, but, morals are religiously derived admonitions and prescriptions. They are considered to be transcendent and handed down by a super-ordinate spiritual entity, acceptance of them is based on faith. Norms are expectations and rules of a specific social system (e.g., family, group, organization or society). They denote what is considered to be appropriate/acceptable behavior within that system; adherence is based on affiliation, membership and affinity. All this said, ethical principles are often adopted as morals and norms.
[21] I initially developed this model as a teaching tool for my graduate-level courses in organization behavior and management. It condenses and facilitates the application of a number of hard-to-grasp ethical theories. When I started using the pyramid in board retreats, directors said it made sense.

The Ethical Pyramid

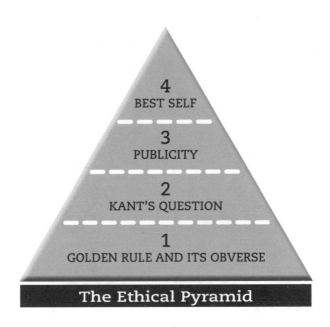

4
BEST SELF
— — — — —
3
PUBLICITY
— — — — — — — —
2
KANT'S QUESTION
— — — — — — — — — —
1
GOLDEN RULE AND ITS OBVERSE

The Ethical Pyramid

- This model lays out four ethical tests that are progressively stringent.

- For a decision/action your board is contemplating, subject it to each of the tests in sequence.

- (1). Does the proposed decision/action abide by the Golden Rule and its obverse? That is, in making a decision or undertaking an action are we: doing unto others as we'd like done to us; and/or are we not doing unto others that which we wouldn't like done to us? These ethical principles are based on the notion of positive and negative equity: "What goes around should come around." It's indefensible, unjust, unfair and illogical to do something to another party that we wouldn't tolerate being done to us.

- (2). Kant's[22] question asks: Are we willing to make the premise on which the decision/action is based into a universally applicable principle? Here's an example: Say you don't declare cash revenue on your personal income tax return. Is this ethical? It is if you'd be willing to extend the premise and allow everyone else to do like-wise; it's not if you wouldn't.[23]

- (3). How would we feel if others were aware of the decision/action, in addition to the intentions and motivations underlying it? Would it withstand public scrutiny? That is, if a transcript of the board's deliberation of the matter were published on the front page of the local newspaper, would we be proud?[24]

- (4). Is this decision/action compatible with the image we have of our organization and board at its very best? Are we holding ourselves to the highest standard demanded of those entrusted with our community's health and well-being?

Organizational ethics begins with your board setting and demonstrating the right tone at the top.

Directorship

- Ethics is something rarely discussed openly and explicitly

---

[22] Immanuel Kant (1734-1804) was one of the "founding fathers" of the deontological school of ethics, holding that the relative goodness of decisions/actions is determined by the nature of the process employed to arrive at them (rather than intentions or outcomes *per se*).

[23] This simple principle can be applied to all types of decisions and actions. Ethical behavior (from Kant's perspective) should increase the probability of human survival by reducing social chaos. Being willing to "extend the premise" on which a contemplated decision/action is based beyond the self, as an ethical test, does this. Kant's principle is a more general and sophisticated specification of the golden rule.

[24] *Anecdote:* As Associate Director of UCLA Medical Center (from 1975 to 1986), I had the honor and pleasure of working for a phenomenal man: Baldwin Lamson, MD. "Baldi" had an overarching principle he demanded his executive team heed in conducting business: "We'll say or do nothing that we wouldn't be proud to see reported on the front page of the *Los Angeles Times*." And he walked the talk.

in boardrooms. Your board might take some time at a meeting or retreat to talk about features of the ethical climate/ culture it wants to build and sustain, and the ethical expectations it has for itself and directors.

- Suggest that your board discuss how it could employ the pyramid model to assess the ethical quality of proposed decisions and actions. It's probably wise to restrict a formal analysis to only the biggest and most important issues and deals.

- As a director, I apply these ethical tests to most important matters I'm asked to consider and vote on in the boardroom. I find it to be a useful "gut check."

- Given the current crisis of confidence regarding organization and governance ethics, your board should seriously consider formulating a code of conduct for directors and officers. If you want some advice and background materials, consult:

  - *Developing a Code of Conduct for a Corporate Board of Directors – A Map*; Ethics Resources Center, www.ethics.org/resources/articles-organizational-ethics.org.

  - The Business Roundtable; Institute for Corporate Ethics, www.corporate-ethics.org.

- For more depth on ethics in the boardroom, I recommend: *Ethical Governance In Health Care – A Board Leadership Guide for Building an Ethical Culture*, by Roger Ritov, et. al; *Emerging Standards for Institutional Integrity: A Tipping Point for Charitable Organizations*, by Barry Bader, et. al; and *Organizational Ethics in Health Care*, by Philip Boyle, et. al.

Maxim 28

Do governing work only in the boardroom.

The only appropriate time and place for doing governing work is during meetings in the boardroom. This seems too obvious to mention, but I see this maxim violated all the time. For example:

- An important issue is avoided, glossed over or tabled, then it's dealt with by a few powerful directors in the parking lot after the meeting has ended.

- A controversial proposal is on an upcoming agenda. Several days prior to the meeting, the chair convenes her kitchen cabinet *via* telephone conference call to form a consensus so the board's leadership can lock arms and facilitate acceptance of the proposal by other members when it comes up for discussion and vote.

Boards are social systems; accordingly, they're subject to political dynamics. But, when driven by them, board cohesiveness ... and ultimately their performance/contributions ... is compromised.

What I call "parking lot governance" is counter productive for several reasons. First, it's divisive. Factions and cliques are created within the board. Second, it's centrifugal; director energy and attention is fragmented, not focused. Third, it increases the probability of minority rule; a small group comes to agreement about something and then "steamrolls" other directors before they can get their act together.

- Most governmental boards have policies (or are subject to so-called "blue sky" laws) that prohibit more than three directors from meeting in private to discuss governance matters. This is overwrought and difficult to enforce. However, I recommend that your board: discuss the problems of "parking lot governance" and clarify expectations that governing be done only in the boardroom.

- Avoid being drawn into significant outside-the-boardroom deliberations. Indeed, when approached, suggest the appropriate place to hash-out such matters is during meetings with all directors present.

- Don't let this maxim inhibit you from calling, or meeting with, other directors to clarify issues or seek information.

MAXIM 29

STROKE.

Behavioral scientist and management guru Kenneth Blanchard[25] often speaks about the power of strokes (positive feedback) in interpersonal relationships and groups. They're the ultimate rewards in all human systems; someone noticed, cared enough and made the effort to say something positive. The power of such "warm fuzzies" are increased because they're rare in most professional settings.

Directorship

- In a board meeting when a director colleague makes a point/observation you find particularly helpful, thoughtful or enlightening, say so. There's no need to make a big deal of it; your gesture will be heard and appreciated. As a side benefit, this type of behavior (and the positives that flow from it) will catch-on in the boardroom.

- I make it a practice to shoot-off notes to the chair, director colleagues, CEO, and executive team members when they've done or accomplished something outstanding. In the past I sent handwritten notes; I now e-mail. I look for opportunities to do this when the occasion is appropriate: a great report/presentation, major project completion, election to an office in a professional/trade association, winning an award, personal accomplishment, etc. Keep these notes personal and never copy them to others.

- Keep in mind that strokes too often given can be perceived as self-serving and lose value over time.

---

[25]   Blanchard is the author of such hits as *The One Minute Manager* and *Gung Ho: Turn On the People in Any Organization.*

Maxim 30

Don't make individual requests of the CEO and executive team members.

This is based on one aspect of *Maxim #11*, noting that directors have no individual authority or power. As a general principle: requests directed to the CEO and other executives should come from the board; typically the chair, not individual directors.

If this sounds a bit draconian, think for a moment about the consequences if the principle isn't heeded. The CEO and executives receive a flurry of uncoordinated, idiosyncratic, un-prioritized and potentially conflicting requests that would require their attention and time. The result is chaos.

Directorship

- Consider discussing the "no individual director requests principle," and formulating a board policy regarding it. If this is too formal for your board's taste, it should (at a minimum) agree to the notion as an expectation/norm. Doing so makes it a bit easier for executives, when approached by individual directors with requests, to say: "I'm not sure this is a good idea. Remember the board's 'running rule' regarding this."

- There must be exceptions. The most significant are relationships between board committee chairs and their executive team member counterparts. For example, the chair of the finance committee must be able to make requests of the chief financial officer. In doing so, however, one must keep in mind that it's easy to create a lot of work for others by making requests that are not well thought out.[26]

---

26   *Anecdote:* When Associate Director of UCLA Medical Center, I was having lunch with a staff assistant who reported to me. I casually mentioned that it would be nice to have an analysis of _____. Two weeks later she sent me a beautifully researched and written 30 page report which I neither really needed nor wanted. All I was doing during our lunch was "thinking out loud." The lesson learned, and which I've never forgotten: Be carefully what ya say, because people listen and take you seriously.

Maxim 31
BE PREPARED TO VOTE NO.

After you've processed all the data/information, entertained the recommendations of board committees and management, listened to your colleague directors and weighed the needs/interests of stakeholders ... always be prepared to cast a no vote. Lee Iacocca (former President/CEO and Board Chair of Chrysler) once said: "The biggest organizational debacles have been prevented when a few directors had the courage to go against the crowd and vote 'no.' Far too often, management's plans and proposals move through boardrooms like grease through a goose." Where were the no votes in the boardrooms of Enron, Tyco, Global Crossings, AHERF, HealthSouth and UnitedHealth Group? The answer: There weren't any. Not one!

I've seen directors who wouldn't, under any circumstances, vote no. They'd ask tough questions, raise objections, and express dissenting opinions; but when the "chips were on the table," they just didn't have the fortitude, strength of conviction or courage to go against the flow.

Directorship

- Full/open discussion and deliberation among members of a well functioning board will typically precipitate healthy consensus, thus making the need for no votes rare.

- When you cast a no vote:

  - provide your rationale for doing so, completely and specifically,

  - make sure your statement is captured in the minutes, and

- when the minutes are circulated, check to ensure the rationale underpinning your vote is fully and accurately reflected; if it's not, request the minutes be amended.

- For really important issues on which I've cast a no vote, I make it a practice to file a memo with the board chair laying-out my rationale, requesting it's appended to the minutes.

MAXIM 32

ARGUE IN THE BOARDROOM, LOCK ARMS WHEN YOU LEAVE IT.

Truly great governance is characterized by vigorous/robust discussion, deliberation, questioning and debate in the boardroom. However, once votes have been cast, directors must unequivocally and unanimously support the board's decision; no minority reports, no carping, no dissention. To be effective and empowering, boards must speak with a coherent voice. To do otherwise, causes confusion and precipitates conflict.

This is a hard maxim for many novice, and some experienced, directors to accept/heed. But, it's critical for ensuring optimal board functioning and governing effectiveness. The best way to demonstrate this is by considering the alternative: Each time your board makes a significant, tough, and contentious decision, a few directors who voted no actively express their descent to various constituencies ... perhaps even suggesting they shouldn't support it. Such behavior is, frankly, mutinous and undermines a valuable board asset: one focused and forceful voice.

Directorship

- Once a vote has been cast, support your board's decision even if you disagree with it. Boards exercise authority through consensus or majority vote. Once your board has made a decision, you have no legitimate and credible dissenting voice as an individual director.

- If there are too many issues where your conscience does not allow you to support the board's decision, resign and speak your piece.

Maxim 33

Don't engage in personal financial dealings with other directors or executives.

The relationships among directors/executives are complex enough; they don't need to be made more so by the potential difficulties introduced through personal financial dealings. Illustrations (to cite only a few) include: any type of business partnership, whether you have a significant or minority interest; joint ownership of a physical asset such as a boat or vacation property; pooling of funds for making investments; taking investment advice, particularly involving a significant outlay of funds; receiving discounts (not generally available to the public) on goods or services purchased; and extending or receiving loans.

Here are some of the problems:

- First, they will (if only subtly and at the margin) compromise your objectivity in dealing with the person with whom you have a financial relationship.

- Second, the relationship could be perceived as suspect and demonstrate a lack of good judgment, even if legally appropriate. Boards, particularly those of nonprofit organizations, are being subjected to standards of behavior by the public and press that transcend the "letter of the law." In this regard, refer to *Maxim #27* and the ethical pyramid: Would such a relationship pass the test of publicity?

- Third, if the financial deal goes sour, there's nowhere to hide. You must continue interacting with the colleague director or executive, and this could be problematic.

- If you're being considered for board membership and have such dealings, disclose them upfront at the earliest stage of the process. My advice is: disentangle yourself from them; and, if you can't or don't want to, consider withdrawing.

- If you're a director and have financial dealings with other board members or executives: disclose them immediately; disentangle yourself from them; and, if you can't or don't want to, considerer resigning.

- Such relationships, and the potential problems they pose, are off the "radar screens" for most boards. You may not agree with my conservative approach. That's OK. Suggest that your board discuss the matter and then formulate a policy regarding it. Some questions you might address are:

  - Should such a restriction be imposed? Some argue that since it's not legally required, there is no reason to do so. If problems arise, they can be handled like any other limited conflicts-of-interest (see *Maxim #25*). Personally, I don't think this does the job. The reason: rarely do these type of relationships pose direct material conflicts regarding specific issues coming before the board. They're always subtle, nuanced and "under the waterline."

  - Who should be targeted? Directors are self-defining. Executives will have to be explicitly specified. I recommend employing the definition of "officers of the corporation."

- Should thresholds be created to eliminate "minor/insignificant financial transactions and relationships?" The answer is an obvious "yes," but this is difficult to specify and codify.

- Here's the big conundrum: Should exceptions (either general or specific) be made for physician directors in their dealings with each other? Most doctors are involved in financial relationships with other physicians. Some are very broad in scope (such as practice partnerships, medical groups/corporations, IPAs and joint ventures). Hence, imposing a "no financial interrelationship policy" on physician directors could significantly restrict the pool of board candidates. My recommendation is to assess, and entertain exempting (if warranted), specific types of financial relationships at the time a physician is being nominated or re-appointed to the board.

MAXIM 34

NEVER DO NON-GOVERNANCE WORK FOR THE ORGANIZATION.

As a director, you should never perform non-governance (managerial or operational) work for the organization.
Here are a few examples:

- The organization is considering purchasing a piece of commercial real estate to build a new outpatient surgery center. It needs the property appraised and, outside the boardroom, this is your line of work. The CEO asks you to render an opinion.

- After months of analysis, the management team has narrowed a list of potential providers for an integrated information system (IS) to three vendors. You are a senior partner in a nationally recognized IS consulting firm, and management would like your assistance in making the final choice.

- [This one is real, involving me.] You're a governance consultant and a board on which you serve has decided to undertake a thorough governance assessment and then (based on the results) redesign its structure, functioning, composition and infrastructure. The chair gives you a call and says: "We'd like you to undertake this project. You know the organization and the board. We've all read your books. I can't think of a better person to do this."

My recommendation: Resist the natural inclination to be of assistance. Heed this admonition, even if you're not compensated.

Directorship

Why you shouldn't lend a hand:

- First, in doing so, you cross and blur the line between governing and managerial/operational work. This could compromise your objectivity and relationships with the CEO, executive team and colleague directors.

- Second, it's difficult (if not impossible) to be a "prophet in your own house."

- Third, if you provide bad advice or make a mistake, your role as a director could be jeopardized for some time to come.

- Fourth, if you are compensated, doing non-governance work for an organization on whose board you serve can raise what are called "inurnment issues." It's best to check with counsel regarding this.

M AXIM 35

KEEP YOUR PERSONAL RELATIONSHIP WITH THE CEO AT ARMS-LENGTH.

I've seen this too often: The CEO recommends friends for board appointments, or, over time, several directors become CEO intimates. This is always a road to potential problems for directors, the CEO and the board as a whole.

Clearly, well-oiled professional relationships between directors and the CEO are critical for effectively/efficiently functioning boards. The key, however, is the nature of these relationships; always professional, never intensely personal. When there's a personal relationship, an appropriate/healthy boundary is hard to draw and maintain over time.

As a director, you will be required to participate in:

*   assessing the CEO's performance/contributions, adjusting the compensation package and (in rare instances) terminating his/her employment relationship with the organization, and

*   reviewing and approving/disapproving proposals and plans forwarded to the board by the CEO.

Such tasks require a degree of objectivity and distance difficult to achieve when you have a close relationship with the CEO; even with the best intention of keeping friendship out of it.

Directorship

*   If you are approached to serve on a board where you're a close personal friend of the CEO, walk away. If you accept, sooner or later your service will be compromised; in

fact, or in the perceptions of your director colleagues. Seek safer ground. Other opportunities for board service will come your way.

- If you're a presently serving director, keep your relationship with the CEO cordial, friendly but strictly professional. If you want to deepen it, resign from the board and do so.

- It's a good idea to maintain only professional, and never personal, relationships with executive team members.

MAXIM 36

PROVIDE THE CEO ADVICE AND COUNSEL WHEN ASKED, BUT BE CAREFUL.

As a director, you may be occasionally sought-out by the CEO and asked for advice and counsel. It's natural for a CEO to consult individuals who are familiar with the market/competitors, in addition to the organization and its strengths/weaknesses. Directors can be helpful sounding-boards. But there are potential potholes and pitfalls.

Directorship

- Recognize in these situations that you're acting as a counselor, not a director *per se*. Advice given can be either taken or rejected. The "running rules" are totally different than in the boardroom.

- Explore the CEO's motivation/intention regarding their advice seeking. Do so by simply asking, then probe a bit. I'm always wary about someone seeking my input in the guise of softening me up regarding a proposal "coming down the pike" or trying to find out where I or other directors stand on an issue. When I sense this, I proceed cautiously or back away.

- I prefer to talk about only substantive issues in such sessions; never discussing, or rendering opinions about, board process/politics or director personalities. Doing the latter could put me in a very uncomfortable and untenable position with colleagues.

- Recall *Maxim #28*, "Do governing work only in the boardroom." A CEO who meets too often with directors (individually or in small groups) to seek their advice is playing with fire. This can create favorites/cliques, be divisive and will eventually fragment a board.

- All this said, there are times when a CEO really needs someone to talk with. It's lonely at the top and an informed, one-on-one, director perspective can be invaluable.

M AXIM 37

BE PREPARED TO LEAD.

Great governance requires great leadership. In this regard, I believe threre is a problem, if not a crisis, brewing. Chairing a nonprofit healthcare organization board demands a huge commitment of time and effort. Unfortunately, it's a role fewer directors are willing or able to undertake. The most able are recruited to boards, but they are also the busiest people. More and more boards are experiencing difficulty getting directors to step-up and assume the role of board chair. As an aside, commercial corporations don't face this problem, as most chairs are their organizations' presidents/CEOs. I don't feel it's wise to move in this direction,[27] but it may become a forced choice or increasingly attractive option in some circumstances, absent a pool of directors who volunteer to lead.

Directorship

- Think seriously about arranging your personal/professional affairs so you could entertain the possibility of assuming the chair role if asked and when the time is right.

- Most boards do no/little chair succession planning. This is required so that directors can make their plans and subsequently transition into the position. Encourage your board to think about its needs, the pool of potential candidates, who might be encouraged to serve and when.

- Boards must increase the attractiveness and "do-ability"

---

[27] Combination of the president/CEO and board chair roles concentrates too much authority and power in one position. Commercial corporations have been increasingly adopting the nonprofit model (albeit slowly), separating the two roles.

of the chair position. Two things warrant serious consideration:

- increasing staff and other resources to support effective/ efficient execution of the role. [Critical here is adequate board/chair staffing. If you'd like to see an illustrative *Board Coordinator Position Charter*, log-on to www.BoardFood.com, go to the navigation aids page and download the document.]

- compensating the chair, irrespective of whether other directors are paid. [This is a contentious issue fraught with challenges. If you'd like to have the briefing paper, *Director Compensation in Nonprofit Healthcare Organizations*, log-on to www.BoardFood.com, go to the navigation aids page and download the document.]

• Yes, the chair role is demanding … but the rewards are many and significant. I've stepped up to the plate several times and have never regretted doing so. The opportunity to exercise leadership in one of the community's most important institutions is priceless.

M AXIM 38

BE A GOOD BOARD AND ORGANIZATIONAL CITIZEN.

In the Disney movie, Bambi was told by his mother: "If you don't have something nice to say about someone, say nothing at all." Great advice for board members. As a director, what you say carries great weight. Don't say anything ... by design or accidentally ... that disparages or discredits the organization, management, the board, colleague directors, members of the medical staff, employees, etc., etc. Indeed, you're expected to be an organizational advocate and supporter; seize every opportunity to be one.

Actions speak far louder than words. Show up for a respectable number of fundraisers, recognition dinners, golf tournaments and silent auctions. Participate in events where director attendance is requested and expected: employee pancake breakfasts, nurse appreciation days and new employee orientations.

Most important (if possible), use YOUR hospital and its medical staff as your source of healthcare. The directors of General Motors shouldn't be driving Hondas.

Directorship

- The stuff of this maxim is often viewed as peripheral to being a successful director. It's not. If you are perceived to be unsupportive of the organization on whose board you serve, your effectiveness will be compromised.

M AXIM 39

PRIOR TO THE CONCLUSION OF EACH TERM, ASSESS YOUR PERFORMANCE AND CONTRIBUTIONS.

The boards of virtually all organizations (with varying degrees of diligence and quality) evaluate the performance and contributions of their CEOs. However, it's been estimated that only 15 percent of *Fortune 500* boards assess individual directors. My experience suggests the figure is far less for nonprofit healthcare organizations.

If your board doesn't have a director assessment mechanism in place, suggest it be considered; I won't go into the specifics here as they've been discussed in *Getting to Great: Principles of Healthcare Organization Governance*, by Dennis Pointer and James Orlikoff (Chapter 7, pp. 126-128).

But, don't wait. Take the "bull by the horns" and assess thyself.

Directorship

- If you'd like to have an illustrative *Director Self-Assessment Instrument*, log-on to www.BoardFood.com, go to the navigation aids page and download the document. Your board can use this inventory as a point of departure for designing a process. It also provides a check-list for doing your own personal appraisal.

- Several months prior to the conclusion of your term, do some reflecting. Take out a sheet of paper and list your greatest strengths and weaknesses from two perspectives: contributions and accomplishments (what you've done) and behaviors in the boardroom and committees (how you've gone about it). Be honest with yourself and focus on specifics (vague generalities will get you nowhere). Contrast yourself with several high performing and contributing directors. Most important, compare yourself with what you could/should become at your very best.

- Next (and this takes some courage) schedule time to talk with the board chair or a director you most admire and whom you are likely to get straight feedback. Share your self-assessment with him/her. Seek their observations, perspectives and input.

- Based on your self-assessment and the feedback received, rough-out an action plan for the next year to improve your director performance and contributions. It need not be elaborate, but must be specific and concrete. I recommend keeping the list short: six to eight things you're highly committed to doing different and better.

MAXIM 40

ENJOY THE JOURNEY AND HAVE FUN.

Serving on a nonprofit healthcare organization board should be one of your most rewarding and enjoyable experiences, in terms of both what you give and receive. You've been accorded a wonderful opportunity to:

- learn about a very interesting industry/organization, the provision of healthcare services and the medical profession,

- assume a leadership position in one of your community's most important institutions,

- make a difference on behalf of stakeholders, aligning the organization's resources/capacities with their needs and interests, and

- work with a group of talented, committed and connected individuals.

Take full advantage of, and revel in, this experience!

Directorship

- Over the years, I've come to realize that to really make a contribution and get the most out of board service (two sides of the same gold coin), the critical ingredient is being willing/able to invest the necessary time and effort. Frankly, there've been occasions when I was stretched thin. Too much teaching/consulting/writing and sitting on too many boards. The lesson: arrange your affairs so you can fully engage with the board on which you serve … and (to borrow an admonition from Oprah Winfrey), "Suck the bone marrow from this experience."

• Board service should be empowering and up-lifting … the operative term is FUN. Having fun is a powerful and essential motivator. Not having fun is debilitating, making board work drudgery. We all have an internal meter that registers a "fun quotient" for every activity in which we're involved. Pay attention to it, particularly when it's low for any significant period of time.

Anecdote: Some time ago I had served on a board for five years (most of the way through my second of three terms). The organization was strategically, operationally, and financially fit and well managed. Plus it was doing important work in an area of interest to me. My colleagues were first-rate and I always looked forward to our quarterly meetings. When several new directors, very high-powered CEOs in parallel industries, were elected, the climate changed dramatically. I won't go into the specifics, but the boardroom became increasingly adversarial and hostile. I shared my concerns with the CEO, chair and several lead directors. They agreed with my observations, but were unwilling to raise the issue with the new directors or board as a whole. My fun meter was registering lower and lower, So, at the end of my second term, I decided to resign.

• If you're having fun, spread the joy. Let the chair, colleague directors and the CEO know it (recall *Maxim #29*, "Stroke"). Often we're too reserved about such things.

Anecdote: When writing this maxim, it hit me that I wasn't practicing what I was preaching. Several weeks later, at a meeting of a board on which I presently serve, I took a few minutes and expressed: what an honor it was to be a member of this crew; how much I was learning from everyone; how I valued our interpersonal relationships; and the importance of the work we were doing together. This prompted other directors to share their feelings; it was a meaningful and empowering experience.

I hope you've found this little book worthy of your valuable time, and the 40 maxims useful for improving the quality of your directorship plus getting the most out of serving on a nonprofit healthcare organization board.

Now (using NIKE's trade-marked tag line), "Just do it" ... keeping in mind Yogi Berra's words of wisdom: "Ninety percent of this game is half mental."

References and Resources

Bader, Barry, et. al; *Emerging Standards for Institutional Integrity: A Tipping Point for Charitable Organizations* (San Diego, CA: The Governance Institute, 2006).

Beazley, Sara, et. al (editors); *The U.S. Health Care Delivery System: Fundamental Facts, Definitions and Statistics* (Chicago, IL: AHA Press, 2007).

Blanchard, Kenneth; *Gung Ho: Turn On People in Any Organization* (New York, NY: William Morrow and Company, 1998).

Blanchard, Kenneth and Spencer Johnson; *The One-Minute Manager* (New York, NY: William Morrow and Company, 1982).

Board Roles and Responsibilities: Elements of Governance (La Jolla, CA: The Governance Institute, 2002).

Boyle, Philip; *Organizational Ethics in Health Care* (San Francisco, CA: Jossey-Bass Publishers, 2001).

Bujak, Joseph; "How to Improve Hospital-Physician Relationships" *Frontiers of Health Services Management* (Winter, 2003); pp. 3-51.

Building an Exceptional Board: Effective Practices for Healthcare Governance – Report of a Blue Ribbon Panel (Chicago, IL: Center for Healthcare Governance, American Hospital, 2007).

Burns, Lawton R., et. al; "The Fall of the House of AHERF: The Allegheny Bankruptcy – A Chronicle of the Hows and Whys of the Nation's Largest Nonprofit Health Care Failure," *Health Affairs* (January/February, 2000); pp. 7-41.

Carver, John; *Boards That Make A Difference* (San Francisco, CA: Jossey-Bass Publishers, 1990).

Chait, Richard, et. al; *Governance as Leadership: Reframing the Work of Nonprofit Boards* (New York, NY: John Wiley and Sons, 2005).

Chang, Richard and Kevin Kehoe; *Making Meetings Work! A Practical Guide to Shorter and More Productive Meetings* (San Francisco, CA: Jossey-Bass Publishers, 1999).

Charan, Ram; *Boards that Deliver* (San Francisco, CA: Jossey-Bass Publishers, 2005).

Christianson, Jon, et. al; *Reinventing the Patient Experience: Strategies for Hospital Leaders* (Chicago, IL: Health Administration Press, 2007).

Cohen, Norman; *The Mentee's Guide to Mentoring* (Amherst, MA: HRD Press, 2005).

Dyer, William G., et. al; *Team Building – Proven Strategies for Improving Team Performance* (San Francisco, CA: Jossey-Bass Publishers, 2007).

Entin, Fredric, et. al; *The Board's Fiduciary Role: Legal Responsibilities of Health Care Governing Boards* (Chicago, IL: Center for Healthcare Governance, American Hospital Association, 2006).

Ensher, Ellen and Susan Murphy; *Power Mentoring: How Successful Mentors and Protégés Get the Most Out of Their Relationships* (San Francisco, CA: Jossey-Bass Publishers, 2005).

Gardner, Karen (editor); *The Excellent Board I* (Chicago, IL: AHA Press, 2005).

Gardner, Karen (editor); *The Excellent Board II* (Chicago, IL: AHA Press, 2008).

Griffith, John R. and Kenneth R. White; *The Well-Managed Healthcare Organization*, sixth edition (Chicago, IL: Health Administration Press, 2006).

Hawkins, Charlie; *First Aid for Meetings* (Wilsonville, OR: Book Partners, 1997).

Holm, Craig; *The Next Generation Physician – Health System Partnerships* (Chicago, IL: Health Administration Press, 2000).

Jennings, Marrion (editor); *Health Care Strategy for Uncertain Times* (San Francisco, CA: Jossey-Bass Publishers, 2000).

Kaufman, Kenneth; *Best Practice Financial Management: Six Key Concepts for Healthcare Leaders* (Chicago, IL: Health Administration Press, 2006).

Kirkpatrick, Donald; *How to Conduct Productive Meetings* (Alexandria, VA: American Society for Training and Development, 2006).

Lee, Fred; *If Disney Ran Your Hospital: 9½ Things You Would Do Differently* (Bozeman, MT: Second River Healthcare Press, 2004).

Leeds, Dorothy; *The 7 Powers of Questions* (New York, NY: Penquin-Putnam, 2000).

Lencioni, Patrick; *The Five Dysfunctions of a Team* (San Francisco, CA: Jossey-Bass Publishers, 2002).

Marion, Robert; *Learning How to Play God* (New York, NY: Ballantine Books, 1991).

Marquardt, Michael; *Leading with Questions* (San Francisco, CA: Jossey-Bass Publishers, 2005).

Morath, Julianne; *The Quality Advantage* (Chicago, IL: AHA Press, 2006).

Parker, Glen and Robert Hoffman; *Meeting Excellence: 33 Tools to Lead Meetings That Get Results* (San Francisco, CA: Jossey-Bass Publishers, 2006).

Permanent Subcommittee on Investigations, Committee on Governmental Affairs, US Senate; *The Role of the Board of Directors in Enron's Collapse* (Washington, DC: US Congress, Report 107-70; July 8, 2002).

Pointer, Dennis D. and James E. Orlikoff; *Board Work: Governing Health Care Organizations* (San Francisco, CA: Jossey-Bass Publishers, 1999).

Pointer, Dennis D. and James E. Orlikoff; *Getting to Great: Principles of Health Care Organization Governance* (San Francisco, CA: Jossey-Bass Publishers, 2002).

Pointer, Dennis D. and James E. Orlikoff; *The High-Performance Board: Principles of Nonprofit Governance* (San Francisco, CA: Jossey-Bass Publishers, 2002).

Pointer, Dennis D. and Dennis M. Stillman; *Essentials of Health Care Organization Finance: A Primer for Board Members* (San Francisco, CA: Jossey-Bass Publishers, 2004).

Pointer, Dennis D. and Stephen Williams; *The Health Care Industry: A Primer for Board Members* (San Francisco, CA: Jossey-Bass Publishers, 2004).

Pointer, Dennis D., et. al; *Introduction to U.S. Health Care* (New York, NY: John Wiley and Sons, 2007).

Reinertsen, James and Wim Schellekens; *10 Powerful Ideas for Improving Patient Care* (Chicago, IL: Health Administration Press, 2005).

Ritvo, Roger A., et. al; *Ethical Governance in Health Care* (Chicago, IL: AHA Press, 2004).

Strachan, Dorothy; *Making Questions Work* (San Francisco, CA: Jossey-Bass Publishers, 2007).

Tyler, J. Larry and Errol Biggs; *Practical Governance* (Chicago, IL: Health Administration Press, 2000).